God's Miracle Among Corruption in Idaho

God's Miracle Among Corruption in Idaho

By

Veverly Myers-Edwards

This edition preserves the original text as published in 2014. New forewords and supplemental front and back matter have been added for this rerelease.

Editorial and publication support for the 2026 rerelease, was assisted by artificial intelligence tools. All content and final editorial judgment remain the sole responsibility of the author.

Published by **Myers-Edwards Publishing**
ISBN (paperback): **979-8-9947756-0-8**
Printed in the United States of America

LEGAL & ETHICAL DISCLAIMER

This book is a work of nonfiction based on the author's personal experiences and contemporaneous records, including medical documentation, correspondence, filings, and official responses available at the time of writing.

All statements are presented in good faith and reflect the author's recollection and documentation of events as they were understood at the time. Individuals and institutions are referenced in connection with documented interactions and matters of public concern.

Legal proceedings described herein were initiated and pursued based on the information available to the author at the time and are presented for contextual and documentary purposes only. This work does not constitute legal or medical advice and does not purport to make findings beyond what is supported by records, sworn testimony, and official materials cited.

The purpose of this book is to preserve a documented record and to examine systemic issues related to patient safety, oversight, and civil rights for public understanding.

DEDICATION

This book is dedicated to my three children, mom, and families who've been impacted by medical negligence and injustice.

Dear Robyn, you endured the loss of your dreams at 13 years old but kept smiling and fighting for your life. I thank God for your strength. Your positive attitude encourages me.

Rodrick and Robert, you two gave me reasons to live and stay focused. You both had to grow up fast and take on a load of responsibilities so that I could assist Robyn. I am so proud of you two for staying focused and not allowing this traumatic event to dictate the outcome of your lives.

To my mom, Shirley V. Myers, who transitioned from this life May 25, 2022, you taught me to stand up for what is right and just; without your love and support, I would not have survived. I am blessed to have had a loving mother like you. You are one in a trillion.

A special dedication to all the patients and families who have endured the loss or debilitation of loved ones due to medical negligence. I pray for your strength in the Lord.

ACKNOWLEDGEMENTS

I thank God for the vision to write this book and for the Holy Spirit which directed and kept me sane through the process.

Sincere gratitude is extended to the following people for their encouragement in completing this book:

My family, there are too many of you to list. So, to all you, I am thankful for everything, whether it was a prayer, or a bill paid on my behalf, I thank you. You're an awesome family.

Linda and Wanda, two amazing Christian ladies who helped edit this book and kept me moving forward, I thank God for your dedication and commitment.

My extended family in Idaho and my friends, I will always remember the love shown towards us during the most traumatic event we've ever had to endure.

Pastor F. Davis, I am so grateful to God that you stopped when I needed direction and took the time to help me.

My Christian sisters who attend the Thursday night Bible study Group at Second Baptist Church, and to the Wailing Women on the Wall Morning Prayer line, thanks for your continued prayers and support.

My Pastor, Kent Hall, and my home church, Shady Grove Missionary Baptist Church, in Memphis, Tennessee, thanks for supporting me and my family. I love you all so much.

If I've left anyone out, to everyone who prayed for us and encouraged us on this journey, I am so thankful for your love and support.

CONTENTS

Foreword – *Robyn Edwards*

It has been seventeen years since I acquired a brain injury. I am thirty-one years old now. One of the most challenging aspects of living with a traumatic brain injury is the lack of appropriate resources and programs designed to support people like me. Too often, individuals with TBI are grouped with populations whose needs are fundamentally different. While I try to take what I can from these resources, it often feels impossible to receive the support I actually need. In those spaces, I don't feel that I am growing.

That gap is what led me to find my voice and break the silence. Out of that need, I recently started a podcast, *Defying Gravity with Robyn O: Living with a Traumatic Brain Injury*, which offers an introspective look into the daily realities of living with a TBI.

Recovery for someone with a traumatic brain injury does not follow a set timeline. Each injury is different, and the complexity of the brain makes recovery unpredictable. Even after seventeen years, I still notice small improvements. I have come to understand that my recovery may take a lifetime and learning to accept that has been part of my journey.

My faith in God played an important role in my recovery. At one point, my family was told that I would never get out of bed again, that I would not be able to eat on my own, and that I would require a feeding tube for the rest of my life. None of those predictions came to pass. While paralysis on my left side permanently affected my gait, I do walk. I eat on my own. I live without a tracheotomy or feeding tube. My faith did not erase the harm that was done or undo the consequences of the stroke, but it sustained me through a recovery that many believed was not possible.

My brain injury was the result of a medical error that could have been avoided. Living with that knowledge has been deeply painful. Growing up knowing that medical institutions were able to alter my medical records and assign false diagnoses left me feeling powerless. It affected my mental health and self-esteem and forced me to confront how easily a person's rights can be violated without accountability.

People often say that I am a miracle. When I regained consciousness, many believed I would never wake up, and survival alone was treated as proof of something extraordinary, but survival came with permanent consequences. The effects of a massive stroke are irreversible, and living with those effects is something I navigate every day.

There are times when I feel discontent, knowing that institutions failed to protect me and instead reduced me to a statistic. As a Black girl growing up in these systems, I often felt unseen and unheard. Some days I feel anger when it seems that no one is listening, and that feeling can lead to depression. These are the hidden consequences of trying to present myself as "normal" while living with limitations that are not always visible. When people judge what they do not understand, it hurts most because these limitations are not something I can control—not my body, and sometimes not even my emotions.

What happened to me was wrong. And given the state of the nation today, amid growing injustice and misinformation, I believe it is time for me to speak. I agreed to write this foreword because, as a Black woman who has lived with the consequences of systemic failure, I believe my voice matters. The records documented in this book stand as evidence of those failures, and I am a living consequence of what happens when oversight does not exist.

I share my story so that the record is not abstract, the cost is not minimized, and the voices of those still living with the consequences of institutional failure are neither ignored nor forgotten.

Foreword – *Veverly Myers-Edwards*

For many years, I questioned God, asking how the events my family endured could possibly work toward any good. I did not understand how witnessing racism firsthand, watching my thirteen-year-old daughter nearly lose her life under the care of a negligent neurologist in Idaho Falls, and exhausting every legal avenue available to us, only to discover that the law did not protect my children or me, could lead to anything meaningful.

When *God's Miracle Among Corruption in Idaho* was first published in 2014, it existed as a living record of harm and institutional failure. I did not write it as a memoir, nor as an appeal for sympathy. I wrote it to preserve documentation: medical records, legal filings, and official responses, because I understood that when oversight fails, records become the only safeguard against erasure.

It is also important to name the context in which this story unfolded. I was a Black mother advocating for my child within predominantly white medical and bureaucratic institutions. In those spaces, credibility is not distributed evenly, and advocacy is often interpreted through the lens of who is speaking rather than what is being said.

My persistence was frequently reframed as disruption, my questions as hostility, and my refusal to accept silence as resolution as a threat to institutional order. These dynamics were not unique to my experience; they reflect documented patterns in how systems respond when marginalized voices demand accountability. To omit this context would be to leave the story incomplete—not because race explains everything that happened, but because it shaped how power responded when harm was named.

Over a decade later, as protections once thought settled began to weaken, I recognized that this record was no longer only about our family. In 2025, amid the rollback of Civil Rights enforcement, the dismantling of diversity, equity, and inclusion initiatives, and renewed efforts to discredit the language used to name systemic injustice, the relevance of this book became unmistakable. What happened to my daughter was not an isolated event. It was the outcome of systems that allowed harm to occur without accountability.

This book documents a pattern of institutional failure: a physician whose actions resulted in catastrophic harm to a child; a lawyer who undermined his own client through distorted records; judicial and regulatory bodies that declined to investigate documented evidence; and state and municipal entities that failed to provide the oversight entrusted to them. Even when evidence of harm was substantial, the system offered no meaningful remedy. For Black families in particular, credibility itself often becomes a barrier to justice.

Debates surrounding DEI, affirmative action, and Civil Rights protections frequently occur far removed from the lived experiences of those most affected by their absence. These protections were not created as abstract ideals; they exist because history has shown that without structural safeguards, harm goes unchecked. The disparities in maternal mortality among Black women, the disproportionate loss of Black lives during the COVID-19 pandemic, and the persistent exclusion of Black professionals from positions of authority all point to the same reality: inequity is not incidental, it is systemic.

As someone who has lived through the consequences of institutional failure, I understand the importance of language. Frameworks such as Critical Race Theory are not weapons; they are tools, ways of identifying patterns that would otherwise remain unnamed. When language is stripped away, so too is the ability to challenge injustice. My own engagement with these frameworks came not through academia, but through witnessing public discourse that sought to silence them. In those moments, I recognized the same mechanisms of erasure my family had faced years earlier.

This book is offered as a case study, one record among many, that challenges claims that systemic racism no longer operates within American institutions. It belongs in libraries, classrooms, and public discourse not as a relic of the past, but as a reminder of the work that remains. While racism may never be fully eradicated, accountability must not be abandoned. Oversight matters. Records matter. And voices grounded in lived experience must not be erased for the comfort of others.

I invite readers to approach this book with care and discernment, understanding that behind every documented failure is a human cost and that preserving the record is often the first act of accountability.

Foreword – *Robyn Edwards (2014)*

In 2007, I had a massive stroke at 13-years-old. I was just starting to realize my abilities and all that I was capable of doing. I feel hurt because the quality of my life will never be the same. Since the stroke, I find it excruciatingly difficult to catch up cognitively and physically. I have granted my mom permission to use my medical records to share my story. I pray that what happened to me never happens to another human being.

-Robyn Oneida Edwards
Costa Mesa, CA 2014

Preface

This edition of *God's Miracle Among Corruption in Idaho* preserves the original text as published in 2014. No substantive changes have been made to the body of the work.

The book is presented as a contemporaneous record—written during and immediately following the events it documents—and reflects the language, evidence, and understanding available at that time. The decision to maintain the original text is intentional. Revising or retroactively reframing the record would compromise its integrity.

Two new forewords have been added to contextualize the material in light of subsequent developments. They are offered to reflect on the long-term consequences of the documented events and to situate the record within current conversations about oversight, accountability, and civil rights.

Readers are encouraged to approach this work not as a retrospective analysis, but as a preserved account of institutional failure—and to consider what it reveals about systems that remain largely unchanged.

Prologue

As I drew closer to completing this book, God began a deep work within me. In September 2013, He led me to examine my own heart—and what I saw was sobering. He showed me how my anger, though justified, was holding me back. I realized that the very people in Idaho Falls, Idaho, who had harmed my daughter and denied us justice, were weaponizing my emotions to cast me as the unstable, grieving mother in denial. Perhaps even worse, they may have portrayed me as deranged. They told countless lies and went to great lengths to misrepresent me—but God knows the truth.

In October 2007, Dr. Erich Garland, a neurologist in Idaho Falls, prescribed a drug to my 13-year-old daughter, Robyn Oneida Edwards, that nearly killed her and left her permanently disabled. Later, I discovered he had altered her medical records to conceal his gross negligence. Even more shocking, in 2012, the attorney who was supposed to represent Robyn's interests used one of those fraudulent records in an attempt to coerce me into dismissing her medical malpractice case.

That moment marked the beginning of a long and disturbing journey through the medical and legal systems of Idaho—a journey filled with betrayal, injustice, and systemic corruption. I reached out to every authority I could: the presiding judge, police, mayor, state medical and bar associations, attorney general, elected representatives, even the FBI and City Council. With few exceptions, I was met with indifference, denial, or outright complicity. Only one voice among them dared to question the integrity of the legal system in Idaho Falls.

As a Christian, I was devastated when God told me to walk away and follow Him instead. It felt like giving up. But He reminded me that His ways are not my ways. While I wanted justice through earthly systems, God had a higher purpose. He would reveal the truth in His time—and on His terms.

Since childhood, I've asked God: "What is wrong with this world?" And time after time, He reminds me: Love people and let Me handle the evil. That's not always easy. I've wanted to fight back, to right the wrongs myself. But time and again, I surrender—because God's way is the only way. Writing this book has been a form of surrender. It has allowed me to let go of anger, to find healing, and to shed light on the dark places within Idaho's legal and medical institutions.

When I began this battle in 2012, God made it clear I would not find justice in Idaho. Still, with every complaint I filed, I hoped—maybe this time someone will listen, someone will look at the evidence. But no one ever did. I became angry and lost sight of God for a moment. Then, in September 2013, the Holy Spirit whispered to me, "You cannot write this book in anger. You must do it as unto Me."

From that moment on, God began reshaping this book—adding, removing, and refining its message. I don't yet know the full scope of His plan for it. I only know that He is its Commissioner.

Looking back, I see clearly: if I hadn't walked through every step of this process—the medical visits, the courtrooms, the denials—I wouldn't have the insight or evidence to tell this story. I wouldn't be able to expose the deeply rooted corruption in Idaho's government and legal systems. These officials believed they were fighting me, but in truth, they were opposing God. He simply used me as a vessel. He knew their hearts—and He knew exactly how they would respond to Robyn and me.

The complicity is staggering. The evidence was always there, yet many refused to examine it—blinded by prejudice, or persuaded by the reputations and influence of those involved. Some of the very individuals responsible may be respected pillars of their communities—Christians in name—who praise God on Sunday but crucify His people in silence on Monday. They thought they could silence me. But God has empowered my voice, not only for Robyn, but for the many families suffering under the weight of medical negligence and judicial failure.

Each year, thousands of Americans die due to preventable medical errors, and countless more are left injured or disabled. The trauma is both emotional and financial—and the system often fails those it claims to protect. Meanwhile, the pharmaceutical industry, worth billions, entices doctors with financial incentives to prescribe their drugs. While many physicians act responsibly, others dispense powerful medications carelessly, often unaware of—or indifferent to—the risks.

This book is my attempt to sound the alarm. It is my cry for justice—not just for my daughter, but for every child and adult who has suffered needlessly. No one should endure what Robyn has. No parent should live through what I have lived through.

In 2007, Robyn was prescribed Zomig, a drug clearly contraindicated for her condition. According to FDA guidelines, Zomig should only be used for diagnosed migraine sufferers—and Robyn had never been diagnosed with migraines. She had visited Dr. Garland once, referred for numbness, not headaches. The drug is not recommended for anyone under 18 and is especially dangerous for patients with possible cerebrovascular issues. Yet he prescribed it, and Robyn was declared brain-dead about October 9, 2007.

The trauma to her brain could not have been more devastating had she been shot. Yet this atrocity was treated as a civil matter—and justice continues to elude us. The barriers have been many. We lived in a community hostile to medical malpractice claims—even when a child is nearly killed. Most patients never file claims because the emotional toll is unbearable. And in Idaho, the lack of integrity within the legal system compounds the pain.

Worse still is apathy. Fighting back feels impossible when powerful professionals close ranks to protect each other. As a minority, I found myself battling three unethical attorneys—one defending the doctor, and two who were supposed to be on our side. And when I turned to the media, I was met with silence. Our story was not told.

Still, I press on. I've written this book as God instructed, striving to be faithful to His vision. I've tried to make it plain and truthful, so that those who read it may run with it—may act on it. My prayer is that this book will spark change, stir hearts, and help end the culture of silence and complicity.

> "I will stand upon my watch, and set me upon the tower, and will watch to see what He will say unto me, and what I shall answer when I am reproved.
> And the Lord answered me, and said, Write the vision, and make it plain upon tables, that he may run that readeth it. For the vision is yet for an appointed time, but at the end it shall speak, and not lie: though it tarry, wait for it; because it will surely come, it will not tarry.Behold, his soul which is lifted up is not upright in him: but the just shall live by his faith."
> —Habakkuk 2:1–4 (KJV)

Parade of Injustice

by Veverly Myers-Edwards

I wonder now, as I am pushed and shoved forward
Did I once stand by the side with averted eyes?
Refusing to look up, can't be a witness
Or maybe afraid that humanity may strike me

As I looked on the crowd, searching for a familiar face
I thought I saw one, but the jerk of a head
Roll of eyes, and a twisted face
They didn't want to be identified

And so onward I moved, and out of sheer exhaustion
I shouted "Don't you see what they've done?"
Then suddenly a lady in the parade scorned me
"What are you doing? They don't care"

"But if they heard me, if they saw me," I said
"Do you think they are blind?" she replied
As I looked around, I saw the signs
Innocent convicted, Guilty set free

Oh, I see a Christian, I see a Christian
How excited I was, and then to my surprise
Their glare vexed my spirit, I started to despair
But the spirit reminded me, Of My Lord, My God

As I looked ahead, the line was thinning
For a moment, I thought we were progressing
As I approached the turn, I saw onlookers waving
Give it up! Let it go! Move on!

People were leaving, they were worn and tired
And I said to the Lord, "Please can I go?"
But instead, he made me a promise
"I will never forsake you"
So, in the parade I stayed.

Chapter 1

God Saw It All

5 Trust in the Lord with all thine heart; and lean not unto thine own understanding.
6 In all thy ways acknowledge him, and he shall direct thy paths.

Proverbs 3:5-6 (KJV)

December 3, 2013, I was compelled to rewrite the first chapter. I thought I was finished. As I stated in the prologue, these individuals have given people a distorted impression of me. I know it, but most importantly, God knows it. Dr. Garland destroyed Robyn's life and attempted to deceive me. G. Lance Nalder and other attorneys connected to the malpractice lawsuit, have attempted to cover it by discrediting me, but God saw it all. This chapter will give information on me and quiet any lies Nalder has told to undermine me.

I am a Christian and an African American-single mother of three. I moved to Moscow, Idaho in August of 2004, after a divorce. When I considered relocating, I took several things into consideration. My oldest son started to withdraw. He went from straight "A's" to "F's" and it was not a gradual fall. The school he attended had lockdowns because kids from other schools were coming over making threats. I did all that I could, even home schooled him one semester. We had all gone through a very rough emotional experience with the separation from their father. They needed down time and so did I.

I decided to relocate to Moscow, Idaho. I was looking for a place where I could feel reasonably safe, and where my kids could level off from the pending divorce. Before I relocated, I attended the University of Memphis. I was awarded a Graduate

Assistantship in Public Administration in 2003. I withdrew from the program after one semester because of the problems at home, which made it impossible for me to meet the demands of the program.

I decided if I was relocating, I needed an occupation with a work schedule similar to the children's school schedule. Consequently, I changed my major to secondary education and enrolled in the University of Idaho's Master's Program in Curriculum Development. When I informed family and friends of my plans to move, I think very few actually thought I was moving.

The decision to move was very difficult. I left behind my very supportive family, a church family that I had known all my life, and several dependable friends. The drive behind the move was the need to get my children out of the line of fire. I refused to allow them to be puns in a divorce war.

A couple of days before we left, I emptied my apartment. I told my children to select three items that they really wanted that could fit into the van. Everything else was either going to the dumpster or into storage. As I was putting furniture and what nots out near the dumpster, a man passed by and asked if he could have the items. His church was having a garage sale, and the proceeds were going towards their building fund. I invited him to the apartment to take whatever he wanted because I needed to get rid of everything.

My Mom decided she was coming with us to Moscow, Idaho. She needed to know where I was taking her grandchildren. Several days before we left, one of her best friends decided she was coming too. It was a tight squeeze, my three children, my mom, her friend and me. I gave away everything but what would fit into the van. We left Memphis, Tennessee, packed like sardines in a Chevrolet Venture, off to a new adventure. That is what I told my children. We were going to explore new things. Since my mom was helping me drive, we stopped a lot more than I would have. She insisted we stop at about 7 pm every night and check into a hotel.

As we drove across the Mississippi River Bridge, crossing into West Memphis, Arkansas, I felt a heaviness within my spirit. I was going to miss my family. Yet, when I considered the emotional stress of the divorce a sense of calm took over my spirit. I knew it would be all right because I also prayed to God and asked Him to meet our needs in Idaho.

By the time we arrived in Nebraska, my daughter Robyn was singing, "I will never see a sunflower again." The boys were quiet. When her older brother was fed up with her singing, he pleaded for her to stop. By the time we entered the mountains, the van was quiet. I think we were all in awe of God's creation. I remember my mom driving down a mountain and the river below gave the illusion we were driving into it. It was beautiful and unnerving until we reached the bottom. I think between my mom and me, we each preferred to be the driver when going through the mountains. She was scared of my driving and I of hers. I actually thought it was a nice trip. Many years passed before my children told me how they hated the long drive, mainly my oldest son. He still prefers to fly than to take the cross country drives.

Moving was definitely a leap of faith. When I arrived in Moscow, I had a four bedroom, empty, apartment waiting. The Saturday morning after we arrived, we arose with a mission, to furnish the apartment on a very limited budget. Our first stop was a church garage sale. I found dishes, a microwave, pots and pans, furniture and several other items. When I asked the price of the items, the lady said "just make a donation." My thoughts, "Thank you Lord." With my challenged budget, by the time I left the church, I had just about furnished the apartment.

I am thankful to the Lord because there were moments when I felt defeated and wanted to give in to my feelings of desolation. But somehow when I turned inward, and blocked out the world, blooms of faith sprouted from the word of God within me. It gave me the strength to stand, hope to overcome, and faith to believe in the impossible workings of God. My experiences with my Heavenly Father have led me to become even bolder in my faith and belief in His word.

After I completed the mandatory classroom courses, I finished the remaining courses online through the University of Idaho. The next summer, we moved to Idaho Falls, Idaho. One of my Moscow neighbors mentioned this was a place of clean living. I visited Idaho Falls, Spring Break of 2005, to look around and find a place to live.

Our first night in Idaho Falls, we ate at a Bar-B-Q restaurant. The food was delicious. The owners were kind and inviting. The owner's wife joined us at our table. She and I talked a while. It seemed as if we had met before. She invited us to breakfast the next morning. While eating breakfast with them, their pastor and his family came in. We met them and my oldest son, and his son became friends. Before I left Idaho Falls to return to Moscow, I had found friends and a church family.

Once we moved to Idaho Falls, we joined New Covenant Ministries Church of God in Christ, where my friend and her family attended. I was active in ministry there. During my membership, I taught Sunday school and assisted with the youth ministry and women's ministry. Robyn and I also choreographed praise dances and sang on the praise team. After a couple of years in ministry, I was licensed as an Evangelist Missionary. My first reaction to the position/title was that it was not necessary. My pastor informed me that I was already doing the work.

The Idaho Jurisdiction of the Church of God in Christ is small but diverse. I will always cherish the love and support extended to my family. When Robyn became ill, several members from Community Church of God in Christ in Idaho Falls, spear headed a benefit for Robyn. New Covenant Ministries and New Hope Church of God in Christ also took part in the benefit. Although I could not attend because I was at Robyn's bedside, I was told by family, co-workers and others who were not affiliated with the church that it was an event they would never forget. One of my co-workers, who volunteered to work the event, said that it was the spirit of the people that made the difference. The African American Alliance in Idaho Falls also provided their support during this time.

Before Robyn's illness, I worked for Idaho Department of Labor in Idaho Falls. I really loved my job, my co-workers and the management team. I worked in the Workfirst Program. The goal of the program was to assist people in finding employment. The opportunity to encourage people and help them rise above their circumstances made up for the low pay. By the time I was near the end of my Master's Program in Secondary Education, I decided I wanted to work with adults.

One of the challenges I found with the Workfirst program, was that finding employment was often an enormous challenge. Many of the employers that offered the opportunity for people to rise above the poverty level seemed out of reach, not only for those without much work experience, but for those with qualifying experience too. For many of my clients, the job search experience was stressful and discouraging, and for me, a challenge to keep them focused.

I took a professional interest in all the participants I case managed. I wanted them to find more than a job. I wanted them to find a career, one they enjoyed. I encouraged them to use the transition to make necessary changes. If they needed to go back to school, this was the time to do it. Some were required to attend the program five days a week. In the mornings, we spent an hour in class. Afterwards, they were required to do job searches and fill out applications. On the Fridays that I facilitated the morning sessions, my morning classes were open forum. Most times the participants used this time to share their experiences and to encourage one another.

When Robyn had her stroke in October of 2007, I had no idea how long I would be off work. I was blessed to have a caring team of co-workers who donated their vacation hours to help me. In February of 2008, Robyn and I left Primary Children's Hospital in Salt Lake City, Utah and returned to Idaho. At that time, I realized that it was impossible to work and help Robyn. So I resigned from Idaho Department of Labor in April of 2008.

Once Robyn was in high school and somewhat situated, I decided to go back to work. In the summer of 2010, I found myself in the same place as many of my past clients in the Workfirst Program, looking for employment. I did not immediately seek to return to the Department of Labor because another agency was awarded the grant which funded the Workfirst Program. Even though the pay was not the best, I loved what I did in that program.

There were times when I became very discouraged at the difficulty in finding a job. I eventually reapplied to Idaho Department of Labor and did not get the position. I was a little discouraged but realized that it was not for me. I was not offended when I reapplied and was not rehired. I applied for a different position. Several months later, when additional positions came open at the Department of Labor, I was offered another position.

In September of 2010, I had an interview with a Federal Contractor at Idaho National Laboratory, for a job that I knew I was well qualified for. It was really difficult to even obtain an interview, and to be seriously considered for a job is an even greater feat. Not that it should be that difficult for a qualified person, but it was. I applied for a Relocation/Recruiter position. After about a month of not hearing from them, I called and inquired about the job. I was told that the managers had already made their selection of candidates for interviews and if I had not been called, then I was not selected. I was all right with this, disappointed, but I had no reason to believe anything unethical transpired.

Well, I also knew a few professional African Americans who worked at the site. I was told about a committee that was formed to monitor/promote the hiring of professional African Americans. So I contacted someone on the committee and forwarded my resume. About a week later, I had a call from one of the persons on the committee. She wanted me to forward my resume to her and inform her of any applications that I submitted through their system.

About a week or so later, while at a physical therapy appointment with Robyn, I received a call from the hiring manager for the Relocation/Recruiter position. She asked me if I was still interested in the position. I said, "yes." I also informed her that I was told that they had made their selection of interviewees. She replied, "I didn't find what I needed in the nine I'd interviewed."

This was exciting for me, an opportunity at a job with mobility that would help me provide for my children. My children and I were ecstatic. This would bring the opportunity to move forward after a traumatic experience and a long three years of rehabilitation for my daughter, and sacrifices from my sons. Finally, it appeared that the sun was about to shine on us again.

The first round was a phone interview; I would have to do well on it to obtain an in-person interview. The phone interview was scheduled the day after I received the call at the therapist's office. I went home that evening and did my research. I was once a Relocation Consultant at a company in Memphis, Tennessee, so I knew what to do to prepare. That evening I accessed the Employee

Relocation Council website. This site has the latest updates and changes in the industry. I knew as a government contractor, their guidelines were more than likely reflective of the federal government, so that is what I studied.

The hiring manager on the relocation side conducted the phone interview. While the position was split between recruiting and relocation, the job requirements specified someone with experience in relocation. While speaking with her, I shared information about the Employee Relocation Council, which she had no knowledge of. That was surprising to me. As we talked, I gave her the Url to the website and she pulled it up as we spoke. She was amazed at the available information. I encouraged her to join, but she said it appeared that a lot of the information was free. The phone interview went very well. I was scheduled for two more interviews the next week.

My children and I celebrated; I had gotten past the first round. Now, on to the second round. Yahoo!!! I studied even more. I even called an old peer that was still working in the industry to give me advice on what to expect. My kitchen table was covered with relocation information. I studied up to the date of the interview.

The first interview was with a male manager. He handled the recruiting side. It went very well. One of the requirements in the job posting was to submit a writing sample. I brought in a ninety-one-page Career Development manual I had to prepare in graduate school. He informed me that I needed to submit the writing sample in my next interview session; however, after flipping through the table of contents, he wanted me to forward him the chapter on Career Development Theories.

After I returned home, the first thing my kids asked me that evening was, "did you get the job?"

The next day, I met with the manager I had the phone interview with and a Human Resource Representative. The HR representative was really nice. The hiring manager was late for my interview. It seemed as if we stood outside her office for at least ten to fifteen minutes. During this time, the HR representative and I shared personal information. I told her about my move to Idaho after a bad divorce and my daughter's illness. She told me about her move to Idaho from California and a niece or nephew she helped out with, because she and her husband did not have kids.

My interview went well. I came to this conclusion after the HR representative told me how well I interviewed and how well my customer service skills served me. She also informed me that I would not have a big learning curve for this job because I have the one piece of experience no one else had, the relocation experience, along with ten years of real estate which was relevant experience. I also have an Education Specialist Degree with a concentration in Human Resources.

Although the interview went well, the hiring manager's behavior during the interview was puzzling. During my interview she brought up the movie, "What Women Want," that features Mel Gibson. I had never seen the movie before and could not see the relevance of it during my interview. She also talked about what men looked for in women. She kept saying they look for "LB." Now, why would this lady do this in my interview?

Before I left the interview, the hiring manager asked the HR representative to give me a benefits package. She requested I look it over and if I had any questions to call the HR representative that scheduled the interview appointments. They also asked questions regarding my limitations. Could I climb steps? Could I lift a certain amount of weight? We went through a list. I acknowledged I had no limitations. They informed me that I would hear from them by Monday of the next week.

I went home so encouraged. My kids asked how it went. I said, "I'm gonna get a job, I'm gonna get a job!" We danced around and shouted with great anticipation. Well, Monday, came and went, and I did not hear anything. On Wednesday morning, the recruiting manager called me and told me they hired someone with more experience and encouraged me to apply for other positions that were coming open. About an hour later, the hiring manager called me. I did not tell her that I had already received a call from the other manager. She stated that she hired someone that spoke better to their processes. She also went on and on about how well I interviewed.

I took a deep breath. I felt a sinking feeling in my gut. I felt like someone had just taken something that was mine. I kept thinking this cannot be. Not that I am so special, but I knew when I saw the job posting that the possibility of someone having relocation experience was probably remote in this area. I also knew that my ten years of real estate experience and degrees-one with a concentration in Human Resources, should have placed me ahead of the others. The HR representative even told me this. There was nothing in the job posting that said the person had to speak to their processes. As a matter of fact, it asked for someone with experience and knowledge of policies and procedures relating to relocation.

When my kids came home from school, the very first question they asked, "Did they call? When do you start? "It hurt me to tell them that I didn't get the job, and to see the disappointment on their faces made my eyes water. I think we all thought this was it, a new beginning. I had promised Robyn that I would re-enroll her in Sylvan Learner Center for Geometry tutoring, if I got the job. I had to pull myself together to keep them focused. "It'll be all right. This wasn't the job for me. I will find something. You all don't need to worry. God has always provided."

I decided to rent the movie "What Women Want." I needed to know how it was relevant in my interview. My children and I watched it together. "Mama, why would the lady mention this movie during your interview?" There were so many scenarios going through my head after watching the movie, I could not answer. Was she trying to tell me that she was not hiring me over someone else? Did she take the information I gave her and decide she did not need me because I had informed her where to go for relocation information and training?

I decided to email the HR representative who was tracking my applications. I told her I felt that I had been discriminated against. She did some research and informed me that they had hired someone internally. This just brought more questions from me. If they had an internal candidate, why did they bring me in after already interviewing nine people? The most puzzling question I had was this, if I had more experience than anyone else, why was I called after the initial phone interviews had closed? The HR representative that interviewed me informed me that no one else had relocation experience. I decided to file a discrimination complaint, but first sent a letter internally through the representative tracking my applications. After sixty days, I decided to file an EEO complaint with the Human Rights Commission.

The Human Rights Commission took my complaint and contacted the Government contractor. After going back and forth, the commission gave us two choices, to try and mediate or I could just opt for an investigation. I opted for mediation. The morning of the mediation, I felt a heaviness in my spirit and with each step I took, it seemed like weights were attached to my legs.

When I arrived at the Department of Labor, I was led to a room. The Human Rights representative came in and introduced herself and informed me that three people had shown up on behalf of the company instead of the one lawyer that I was expecting. I took a deep breath.

'Why wasn't I informed about this? Maybe I would have brought someone with me?"

"Well, Ms. Edwards I didn't know, but I think it makes sense for the manager you filed the complaint against to be here. Is this going to be OK with you?"

"Well, it makes my guards go up because I think it's an intimidation tactic on their part."

"No, No, I don't want you to think that, plus, I will be there to mediate."

I agreed to proceed with mediation. I cannot go into the specifics of the mediation but there are a few things I will discuss. One of the things that came out during our response/rebuttal period was that they changed their reasoning for not hiring me. Instead of sticking to the reason they had given me, which was they hired someone with more experience, it changed to my lack of interviewing skills. During mediation, I asked, "if I interviewed badly, why did the hiring manager and HR representative comment on how well I did during the interview session?" The hiring manager stated that she did not want to offend me.

Well, then someone gave an analogy, "if someone smells bad, you wouldn't tell them."

I replied, "you wouldn't tell them that they smelled good either, would you?" The analogy they gave did not apply in this situation. I did not request their feedback on my interviewing skills. Not that I did not want it, but I did not ask. So if they were going to volunteer the information, why lie to me?

The hiring manager then asked, "do you really want to know why we didn't select you?" Their attorney tried to stop her, but I replied, "No, let her go on. Yes, I want to know."

"Well, during the interview you kept speaking of your daughter's illness. I leaned forward, "Are you implying that I couldn't get through the interview without bringing up my daughter."

"Yes, I am."

"You are a liar. I never even spoke to you about my daughter. The only way you could have gained this information was from the HR representative. Because you were late for my interview, the HR representative and I stood outside your door and shared information about our personal lives."

My belief is the hiring manager brought up Robyn's illness as a way to evoke an emotional response out of me in an attempt to distract me. Their lies were a form of intimidation. I was honestly disappointed that the HR representative took a role in the deception. Their attempts to scare me convinced me even more to press forward for what was right, shining a light on their unfair practices and inhumane behavior. Who would bring up something as devastating as the near death of a child to undermine someone?

At this point, I had made my decision not to settle. When the session ended, the Human Rights representative separated us to start the negotiation process. I felt an even heavier burden now. I knew their intention was to intimidate me, to scare me with the fact that the three people who interviewed me would stick together, using the lie about me speaking of my daughter's illness throughout the interview. That sickened me to the core of my being.

When I was asked what it would take to settle, I quoted an astronomical figure in the millions. The Human Rights representative gave me Idaho's maximum in a case such as this one and I decided to go with that. I also requested my job and any other benefits I had lost. They rejected it, as I knew they would, and I decided not to settle. The Human Rights representative informed me that if I did not settle, I risked losing the opportunity of receiving any compensation. The investigation may find no cause for discrimination. I decided to push for the investigation; even if I lost, at least I knew that I stood for right.

I had a serious problem with the ethics of the employees of this Government Contractor. When I first inquired of the job, I was informed that I had not been selected for an interview. I was fine with this. I had no reason to believe anything unethical transpired. However, when they called me back and took me through a process that I felt was highly suspect of discrimination, I had a problem with it. My belief is, I was brought in just so they could make a quota and say they did consider an African American. I would have preferred not to be a part of their sick process. While there are many arguments as to whether Affirmative Action Laws are useful, what is the alternative? I recall a manager in the meeting telling me that this contractor had met their requirements and had just been audited. She even gave me the numbers.

From my experience with the Federal Contractor, I now know how stressful and discouraging it was for the participants in the Workfirst program. While they were required to find a job, no one took into consideration, a job market where their skills and abilities may have no bearing on their ability to obtain employment. My driving force behind filing the complaint was not only to bring to light what this contractor did to me, but to the many others who attempted, or will attempt to apply and not find success because of the practices of this employer's HR department.

When God places His leaders in positions to expose the corruption of the enemy, we are to stand, and not turn away as if we do not see the injustices. The problem in many instances, is that once comfort sets in, obedience becomes an offense to the senses. Sacrifice, what? No one does that today, right? So even though God purposes our steps, and is the reason for whatever gains we obtain, when we become comfortable, his request may be looked upon as that of the enemy's. Many Christians at this point start to rebuke their blessings because it may cause inconvenience.

I also took part in organizing two women's conferences during 2010 and 2011 in Idaho Falls. The purpose of the women's conferences were to equip women with the knowledge of God to break the strongholds placed on their lives. The theme of the conference in 2011 was "Standing through the Storm." We even had a few shelters that offered to pay for women in their programs to attend.

In the latter part of 2011, a couple of my Christian sisters from another church in the community, asked me to join them in ministering to youth at St. Anthony's Youth Detention Center. I accepted, completed a background check, went through the training and started visiting the Center every fourth Sunday to provide ministry. I was honored and humbled to take a part in such a ministry. While it tugged heavily on my heart to hear the testimonies of the youth, I thanked God for the opportunity to share His word and to speak into their lives.

For me, ministering to others has helped me stay focused while going through my own storms. While I encouraged others, I found hope for myself. I also realized that if I taught something, I needed to live it. I have always taught that the people of God should make a difference wherever they go. Children of God do not bow down to evil. We are not to fit in just to get along with the crowd, nor are we to beat people with the word of God. The way we live speaks for us and when it is time to stand, we can do so. This is the sum of why I stood up against discriminatory hiring practices and a corrupt medical and legal system in Idaho Falls, Idaho. I cannot lead where I am not willing to go.

My experiences in Idaho were mostly pleasant until I met with the unethical practices of Dr. Garland, and found out last year that attorneys G. Lance Nalder and Breck Barton were attempting to undermine Robyn's medical malpractice lawsuit. Additionally, there was the systemic corruption in the medical and legal systems. However in spite of the ruthless and callous actions of the officials, there are some really good people in Idaho Falls. It is unfortunate that the good people are not running the government.

I believe God placed me in this position for a reason. I believe my being led to Habakkuk and the Holy Spirit's revelation to me while I was there, was already purposed by God. These people thought if they undermined me and frustrated me with their dysfunctional processes that I would give up. Yet, it has only added to my conviction that the corruption needs to be exposed to protect others from falling in the same trap.

Taking a stand for justice in Idaho Falls is equivalent to a slave on a southern plantation, standing up to his master and telling him that slavery is wrong. While they cannot publicly hang you and whip you as was done in the South, in their secret chambers they attempt to destroy your character to quiet your voice. I realized after calling one attorney after the other to find help for Robyn, that G. Lance Nalder had sabotaged the Medical Malpractice case. While Dr. Garland destroyed Robyn's life, and Mr. Nalder and his cohorts attempted to hide his negligence by discrediting me, God saw it all.

Chapter 2

God's Miracle

God is our refuge and strength,
a very present help in trouble

Psalm 46:1 (KJV).

During the summer break of 2007, while at her father's house, Robyn experienced a numbing sensation in her leg. When she returned, I made an appointment with her primary care physician. I was very concerned about the numbing sensation because Robyn had not had any medical issues other than a broken bone and a torn ligament. I would lay awake at night wondering what was going on. I had friends and family members try to ease my worry by suggesting it was probably something simple, like a pinched nerve. I tried to make myself believe that, but the spirit within me told me it was more than a pinched nerve.

One morning about 3 am, I was lying in bed talking to God about Robyn and the Holy Spirit led me to go pray over her while she was asleep and to claim victory over whatever was going on in the name of Jesus. My first thought was to just lie in bed and pray, but the Spirit said, "No, go to her and touch her in My name." I got up and I went to her room. I gently placed my hand on her head, prayed, and claimed the victory over whatever was going on in her body.

The Sunday following that experience, while I was sitting in morning services, the Holy Spirit spoke to me again, and said, "If you believe that Robyn is healed in my name, stand before the saints of God and claim it." This made me uncomfortable and I kept thinking Lord these people are going to think I am crazy because Robyn had not shown any signs that anything was wrong. The numbing episodes were few and did not last long.

God knew that I needed a little help. Consequently, the praise and worship leader called on me to do a song that morning which helped to get me up from the pew. The song she requested was, "God Specializes." As I stood before the saints of God, and thought about the song, I began by telling them what God had prompted me to do. I told them how reluctant I was to do it, but being obedient to God, I stood and claimed the victory over Robyn's illness. At that time, I had no clue what was about to transpire in our lives, but God did.

On the night of October 4, 2007, Robyn was taken to Eastern Idaho Regional Medical Center's (EIRMC) emergency room because she had no feeling on her left side and she had a bad headache. Earlier that day, about 12:30 in the afternoon, she had a numbing sensation and I gave her Zomig, the medication prescribed by Dr. Erich Garland. About 2:00 pm, she complained of a bad headache. I gave her ibuprofen because Dr. Garland suggested it during our visit to him on October 1, 2007. Her headache progressed and so did the weakness in her limbs. At about 11 pm or close to midnight, she told me she could not move her left side and had not moved it since earlier in the evening. I had her brother place her in the car and I took her to EIRMC.

Robyn was in the emergency room for nearly twelve hours before she was diagnosed with a stroke.

"Mommy, it really hurts bad," Robyn said.

"The nurse just gave you something for pain, give it a minute to work, OK", I replied.

"Yes, ma'am," she said, as I held her hand inside of mine rubbing it and praying silently. "*Father God please help her*."

"Mommy, it's not helping."

"Robyn when it gets really bad just talk to Jesus. Just try to focus on him." She squeezed my hand tighter.

"Yes, ma'am," she said, as she moved her head from side to side.

"Mommy."

"Yes, Robyn."

"Please don't leave me."

"I promise I won't leave you."

"Mommy."

"Yes, sweetie."

"I love you."

"I love you too Robyn."

"and Mommy."

"Yes."

"Step by step, one day at a time."

"Yes baby, that's what we'll do. Take it step by step, one day at a time." She squeezed my hand even tighter and then drifted back into an unconscious state.

Around noon on October 5, 2007, I was informed that she had a stroke and her condition was critical. Eastern Idaho Regional Medical Center (EIRMC) could not treat her condition. EIRMC made plans to life flight her to Primary Children's Hospital in Salt Lake City, Utah. We were supposed to depart EIRMC at two o'clock that afternoon. The winds were very high that day and there were also thunderstorms in the area. The helicopter EIRMC used could not fly in that weather.

Because her condition was extremely critical, Primary Children's Hospital sent in a small plane. It was a rough plane ride to Salt Lake City. It felt like the wind was playing cat and mouse with the plane. I recall at one point feeling like I was going to be lifted up and thrown, and had it not been for the seat belt, the rocking and jerking motion of the plane would have probably thrust me out.

Under normal circumstances, the plane ride would have unnerved me, but I was still trying to digest the stroke diagnosis. As I bounced up and down, my eyes were fixed on Robyn who was lying on a stretcher that took up most of the belly of the plane. The medical attendant was seated across from her and I was seated in the back of the plane. Robyn was wrapped so tightly in blankets that I could barely see her face. At one point her body started to jerk, but not from the movement of the plane. I started to rise but the seat belt restrained me. The nurse started searching through her medical bag, pulled out something, and with a quick motion pulled Robyn towards her. She placed a bag in front of Robyn's mouth. She glanced at me and made a motion. I realized that Robyn was throwing up. I settled back in my seat.

Over the course of one day, my family's life had changed completely. As much as I wanted to scream, "No, this cannot be happening to her," it was. Robyn, who once ran track, choreographed dances for the praise dancers and sang on the praise team at church, and weeks away from trying out for her high school basketball team, was near death due to a stroke.

Just a month before Robyn's stroke, we had moved into a house. I was tired of renting and wanted to give my children a place of their own. It was a financial challenge, but this was a new beginning for us.

The kids were excited about the move. The house was around the corner from their schools. Robyn's favorite features were the tulips and the roses in the front of the house, and her bedroom. My youngest son was excited about having his own bedroom again. Their older brother was excited because he had the entire basement area to himself. My favorite features were the sunroom off the family room and the huge window in the living room. I made the sunroom my reading and writing area.

I bought a rocking chair and placed it by the huge window in the dining room. Many mornings I sat in the rocker, drank coffee and read my bible. The house had about three thousand square feet of living area. The only feature I had a problem with was the fruit trees in the back yard. I planned to cut them down.

Everything was going well. I had to be at work before the kids' schools started. The older two kids' school started before the youngest one. I was a little uncomfortable with my youngest one being the last one to leave the house. I insisted he call me when he left the house and when he arrived at school. In the afternoon, he returned home first, but Robyn arrived just a little later. We developed a routine that worked out well.

Now a month after Robyn's eighth grade year began and a few weeks before her basketball tryouts, we are being airlifted to Primary Children's Hospital. Robyn has suffered a massive stroke and is in critical condition. "We are about to land," the pilot's voice said over the intercom bringing me out of my muse.

I braced myself for the landing. I tried to wrap my mind around what was happening. Nothing at all made sense to me. Before we left EIRMC, I was told that the stroke was due to a rare condition called MoyaMoya. Days earlier, Dr. Erich Garland, the neurologist in Idaho Falls, Idaho, had diagnosed her symptoms of numbness as a rare form of migraine that caused numbness. By the time the plane landed, my emotions were numb and I was in a state of shock.

——✧——

On the ninth of October the medical team at Primary Children's Hospital requested a meeting with the family. I didn't want to meet. I knew in my spirit that everything within me was about to be tested. I recall the neurosurgeon stating, "We've done all we could but due to the severity of the injury caused by the swelling, she's brain-dead." I watched as my daughter's father placed his hands over his mouth and a soft sob escaped. All eyes were on me. When I looked up, I said, "When I prayed, God put life in my spirit." I'm not sure what was said after that because "*brain-dead*" and "*Robyn is gone*" rang throughout my being. The words entered my ears and slowly attacked every nerve fiber and emotion, and when it hit the soul of my being I silently cried out, "Lord, where are you? Where are you?" I excused myself from the meeting.

As I walked through the hallways, I was vaguely aware of the people standing around. I remember weaving through a crowd, but my mind was still seeking out God. I had no idea where I was going, but I needed a place where I could be alone. I was inwardly searching for that place where God and I met. I needed to contact Him. This was not supposed to happen, and I needed his reassurance.

When I made it to the waiting area it was crowded. So I kept walking. I finally walked into the hallway where the elevators were. It was clear. I sat on a bench facing the elevators. There was a war going on inside my head, despair and hope battling. One thought said, "*Robyn is dead.*" The other said, "*But God said life*." As I sat, with my head in my hands, trying to settle my thoughts, I pulled out my cell phone. The only person I could think to call was my pastor. I knew we were going to need a lot of prayers.

The phone call with my pastor was short. I told him what the doctors said. I told him I would call him back later when I knew more.

After talking to my pastor, my spirit had calmed down a bit. I started to plead my case to God. "Lord, I know you're aware of everything. I've tried my best to raise her according to Your word. I've kept her before You since she entered this world. I know I've failed many times but I've tried my best to be the Christian mother I thought you'd want me to be. I really need you, Lord." As I talked to Him I began to find peace.

I remember hearing a soft voice say "Trust me, only trust me."

"But this is too hard Jesus. I can't do this. They say she's brain-dead."

"I've already given you the victory. Trust Me."

I sat for a while longer. Not sure if I was going crazy or had actually had this conversation with the Lord.

About this time, my sister came around the corner. The meeting with the medical staff was over. She informed me that the doctors were giving us time to consider the next step, and desired to meet with us again later that evening.

My ex-husband was still in the family conference area. I followed my sister back to the meeting room where he was waiting. I took a seat across from him. We both sat in silence for a moment and then he looked up and spoke.

"We've got to decide whether to disconnect her from life support. I can't make that decision," he stated, as tears filled his eyes. "You know if they do the bedside test and conclude that she is brain-dead, they can disconnect life support without our consent."

"No one is going to disconnect her from anything. God really did give me healing for Robyn. We've got to trust that. I won't agree to disconnect her," I replied.

There was a knock on the door. The chaplain entered the room and asked if he could have a moment with us. He was a very compassionate man. He took a seat. Leaning towards me, he began to speak.

"I admire the faith you have in God to heal Robyn, but you do realize that even if he took her, she would still be safe with him," he stated.

"I understand that even if God took Robyn she would be with him, but when I prayed he gave me life and that's what I am standing on," I said.

"What do you want me to pray for?" he asked.

"We need a miracle and that's what we're praying for," I replied.

"Well, that's what I'll be praying for too," he replied.

Before leaving we exchanged hugs. I felt better. At least we had one person on the staff that was praying the same prayer as we were and that believed as we did. Chaplain Jackson and his staff proved to be a very reliable source of spiritual support.

Later that afternoon, we met again with the medical team. Nothing had changed for me. I had made my decision to trust God. The second meeting included a social worker and someone from child life. The team of doctors had reviewed the MRI, CAT Scan, and the EEG. I recall that a female neurologist started the meeting. She began:

"The Robyn you knew is gone." As she spoke, she made a circular motion with her hand before her face. "Her spirit has left. If she lives she'll be in a vegetative state and have no quality of life. The swelling has reached the brain stem which is the control center of the brain. She is no longer able to breathe on her own. If we take her off life support she won't make it through the night. If we leave her on, by the end of the week her major organs will start to shut down and she'll be dead by the end of the week."

My eyes were on Robyn's father. I watched as the pain began to erupt inside him again. He shook his head in disbelief and then placed his face in his hands. The doctor began again.

"Does she have a living will? It's something that you'll need to consider."

"I'm waiting on God. I believe he's going to step in on Robyn's behalf," I stated.

"We'll need to do a bedside test on Robyn. We have it scheduled for Wednesday," she replied.

"Have you ever seen a miracle?" I heard my mom say. "You're about to see one," she stated.

"We have the results of the MRI, CAT Scan and EEG, if you'd like to view them, stated the neurosurgeon.

"Yes, I would," stated Robyn's father.

"No, I don't want to see them," I replied.

I believe the medical team probably thought I was another grieving mother who refused to accept that her child was dead. It did not bother me that they thought I was in denial. I realized at this point that God had given me victory and it was on me to stand and receive it. I decided not to review any more tests. I was not questioning what the test results showed. I was expecting God to show up and work a miracle for Robyn.

Before returning to Robyn's room, I walked back to the benches in front of the elevators and called my pastor. I told him that the doctors said she was brain-dead. His reply to me was, "Sister Veverly what do you want us to pray for?"

"God put life in my spirit, not death. My prayer is for life," I stated.

"Then that's what we'll be praying for too," he stated.

After that call, I went back to Robyn's bedside. It was cold in her room. I entered the room to the sound of a respirator that was assisting her breathing. I watched as her chest rose and fell. She had an IV that dripped liquids into her veins. Another IV dripped medications into an artery. They drilled a hole in the top center of her head and an object stuck out that looked like an antenna. It was connected to a device that read brain activity. She had another device connected to the index finger on her left hand that monitored the blood flow to her brain and her heart rate. A blood pressure cuff was connected to her right arm, which was connected to the same machine that monitored the heart rate and blood flow; it periodically took her blood pressure. The right side of her skull had been removed to relieve pressure on the brain. There was a caution sign above her bed that read "bone flap" and a catheter on the left side of her bed to drain urine.

I walked around to her left side and just stood, still trying to make sense of everything. A long tube also ran into her mouth and back to the machine that was assisting her breathing. The tube was taped around her mouth. Her entire face, head, and neck were extremely swollen, and her mouth was swollen around the taped tube. It was all too much for me. I began to call on the name of Jesus. I then started to rub her down in His name. About this time my sister came into the room, and she stood on Robyn's right side and began to call on the name of Jesus too.

"Jesus, Jesus, Jesus
Jesus, Jesus, Jesus
Savior, Savior, Savior
Savior, Savior, Savior
Healer, Healer, Healer
Healer, Healer, Healer"

We praised and cried out to the Lord until our spirits were satisfied. I remember hearing several people come into the room, but I just continued to call out to the Lord because I needed the peace that only He could give me.

I recall someone touching me. I could feel the hurt and devastation in their spirit, but I refused to turn and receive it. I slowly pulled away. I was at a critical point in my own faith. My spirit was warring with my flesh to believe the impossible.

After my sister and I prayed over Robyn, she left, and I stayed at
Robyn's bedside. She returned a little while later and informed me of her own struggle.

> *" I had to put aside my medical knowledge. I said to myself, we are children of God. Why can't we believe Him for a miracle? I gave family members my medical assessment from what my eyes could see. After touching and agreeing and praying in the spirit with you, the illogical essence of faith (substance of things hoped for, evidence of things not seen) infused my entire being. I called family and church members the second time and stated I changed my mind! I informed them that I was choosing to rebuke the report of the enemy and to believe the report of the Lord. We are a praying family; let's just believe God to perform a miracle," she stated.*

Her response was comforting to me because I knew my reaction to the situation had everyone questioning my emotional state.

Later that evening, before everyone turned in for the night, my mom and I sat in Robyn's ICU room and encouraged each other by searching the bible for scriptures in which Jesus performed miracles. In silence, we found scriptures that supported our situation and passed the bible from one to the other. The one that stuck in my mind was the story of Lazarus. Even though I had heard and read this passage many times, what Jesus did in these verses was more relevant to me now. It encouraged me and supported my position that I could trust Him for the impossible.

At night, I was encouraged by family and the medical team to leave and get some rest. I could not leave Robyn in that condition. I spent the nights in a rocking chair next to her bed. I rocked, sang, prayed and glorified God. I was often reminded of the words she spoke to me before the surgery as she drifted in and out of consciousness. "Step by step, one day at a time."

One of my greatest fears was that Robyn would go into cardiac arrest. The doctors asked if we wanted her resuscitated. Of course, her father and I said, "yes." At night I watched Robyn and took that time to talk to God. I also found myself praying for the other children in the NICU. It was like a jolt to me every time I heard a code blue or saw doctors and nurses rushing to the bedside of another child.

I recall a mother and child being rolled into one of the ICU rooms in the very early hours one morning. The mom was on the stretcher holding the baby. Things seemed OK for a while and then a couple hours later I saw medical staff pouring into the room. I heard a code blue overhead. I saw one nurse start compressions on the child and then another one. I am not sure how much time passed by as I watched, hoping and praying for the mother and child. I remember Robyn's nurse coming to me and gesturing that it was time for shift change. I had to leave. When I returned, the room across from Robyn's looked empty of any life. I realized that my rocker was gone. I asked the nurse about it, and she said they needed it for the family across the hall because the child passed. My heart hurt.

After we were given the news that Robyn would not live through the end of the week, we contacted our family. My other siblings flew in from Memphis. Robyn's father went to Idaho Falls to pick up the boys. He, his friend, and my sister drove to Idaho Falls and brought the boys back. Robyn was swollen so bad I was concerned about them seeing her in that condition.

The child life specialist suggested that she counsel the boys and give them the opportunity to decide for themselves whether they wanted to see their sister in that condition. To prepare them, she took pictures of Robyn to show them. She had dolls that showed the tubes that were connected to Robyn. She explained to them what they would see, and the purpose of the different tubes and machines connected to their sister. My oldest son opted not to see her and the youngest decided he wanted to go in. I think by the time they visited, the swelling in her head had started to decrease a little.

My youngest son wrote a song and a poem for his sister. I posted it on the wall in her ICU room. The poem:

My Sister
You are nice
You are reliable
You are a great sister
You are a great friend
I love you my sister

The song: God is Working

God is working on you
He will heal you if you believe
Praise him, Praise him
Everything will come to pass
If you believe

God will watch over you
He will care
Everything will come to pass in time
God keeps you
God watches over you
God loves you and he cares
He won't let anything happen
If you believe

The bedside test was scheduled for the next day. That night I asked God, "Lord what are you going to do? They're going to perform a bedside test on her." I knew that He was aware of this, but I found peace talking to him about it. Whenever I was told something contrary to what God promised me, I took it back to him.

The morning of the test, I left the ICU for the shift change. In the mornings when I left, her father came in. He was in when the medical team did their rounds. We were all out in the family waiting area when he came through the double doors excited.

"She moved! She moved!" he shouted. "That means she's not brain dead," he exclaimed. That started outburst from all of us.

"Thank you Lord," someone exclaimed.

"Thank You Jesus," another shouted.

"Hallelujah Jesus," I shouted. It went on and on. We must have shouted a while.

Now, I am not quite sure what part of her body she moved. I thought it was her leg, but I have heard different things since then. What I do know is that they lifted one of her limbs and she pulled back, which proved she wasn't brain dead.

Well, it was time for another meeting with the medical team to discuss what that meant. They suggested we not place a lot of hope in her reaction because it was not a purposeful movement. Even if she had some small brain function left, she would have no quality of life if she lived. At this time, we were still told that it was probably better to take her off life support. If she lived, they suggested that we consider putting her in another facility that would provide her long term care. I said "absolutely not, when she leaves, she's coming home to her family." I think most of the staff still thought I was in denial. I was told that if I decided, after taking on such responsibility for her, that I could not provide the care at home, I could always place her in a long-term care facility at a later date.

During the days that followed, Robyn showed small signs of improvement but to the medical staff nothing to be hopeful for. However, I knew that it was God working in her. My ex-husband and I were told she would need a tracheotomy and feeding tube for life. About the end of October 2007, the medical staff realized Robyn was breathing over the respirator. She was now breathing on her own. The doctors still suggested a tracheotomy because several expected her to have another stroke and need to be placed back on the respirator. I did not want it; I knew God was bringing her back.

About the same time Robyn started breathing on her own, she opened her eyes, but she was not conscious. We were told by the medical team not to expect more. One morning, about a week later, Robyn began to scream. The nurse asked Robyn to blink if she understood us. Once for yes, and twice for no. She began communicating by blinking her eyes, but she would not respond to the doctors.

Once her physical and occupational therapists realized she was conscious, they shared jokes with Robyn, and she started responding to them too. She still would not respond to the doctors. I believe they scared her because they talked loudly, as if she could not hear them. I finally asked them to lower their voices. I told Robyn she needed to respond because the doctors did not believe she was conscious. Whenever they did their rounds, she would give them a blank stare.

When the doctors realized she was conscious, there was an onslaught of examinations to determine her baseline. Once the tube was removed from Robyn's mouth, she had a tracheotomy. With the initial removal of the tube, Robyn would not sleep. She would sing and talk all night. Then one day she shared with a representative from Child Life Services that she did not sleep because she was afraid, she would die. It was a while before she would sleep without medication.

There were also tests to determine her cognitive baseline, her mental state then, compared to where she was before the stroke. She surprised the doctors and sometimes embarrassed me. One of the things I realized is that the injury to the frontal lobe of her brain had unleashed a lot of unacceptable language. I immediately started redirecting Robyn. I told Robyn the stroke had opened a lot of gates that needed to be closed. One of the psychiatrist used the analogy of open gates to explain that Robyn's filtering skills had been affected by the frontal lobe injury.

Since I knew Robyn's long-term memory was intact, I instructed her to reflect on what she was taught and encouraged her to think before she spoke. I also asked the medical staff working with her to address the unacceptable language when she used it and redirect her. We gradually made it past the swearing. Thank God!

When Robyn was moved from ICU to the Neuro-science Trauma Unit, several doctors on the medical team informed me that she would have another stroke and surely die. My reply to one of the doctors, "I could have a stroke and possibly die, but no one knows our ending, but God." I never argued with the medical team, even during the very critical days. I was well aware of their opinion of me. Yet, I was never in denial. I knew how bad Robyn's situation was. I sat by her bedside, day in and day out. I watched her lifeless body, and asked God to help me believe. I talked very little because of my own struggles with God's promise to me. I sat by her bedside, rocked, talked to God, and waited for Him to intervene as He said He would.

After the feeding tube was inserted, Robyn wanted to know what it would take for her to eat again. Her speech therapist gave her exercises to do to strengthen her muscles. The feeding tube was inserted the first of November, and by the middle of November Robyn's speech therapist requested a swallow study. On Thanksgiving Day of 2007, my mom brought dinner to the hospital and Robyn ate dressing.

Robyn was slowly regaining her strength, but she was still very weak. She had not sat up without assistance since the stroke. She was transported to therapy in a wheelchair with head support. We had a meeting with the medical team near the end of November 2007. Primary Children's Hospital had a rehabilitation program, but the medical team was not sure if Robyn could meet the rigorous requirements because she did not appear strong enough. I started praying. I wanted Robyn to remain at Primary Children's Hospital. They have a great rehabilitation team.

During this time, my sister and I thought it would be good to place Robyn's favorite scripture on a poster board so that she could see it daily. We requested a poster board from Child Life, and my sister and Robyn put together a poster with pictures of Robyn's progress so far. At the top of the poster was, "I can do all things through Christ which strengtheneth me (Philippians 4:13 KJV).

Robyn and her therapists worked hard. In December, she left the neuro floor and was admitted to the rehabilitation floor of Primary Children's Hospital. Robyn had therapy twice a day with three different therapists: occupational, physical and speech. I remember when Robyn first sat up for five seconds without assistance. That was a major accomplishment. From there it was one triumph after the other. She was slowly but surely moving forward. The staff on the second floor of the Rehab Unit became family to us.

Around Christmas time, one of the doctors from the medical team that managed Robyn's care in the Nuero Intensive Care Unit visited her. This particular doctor was among those who were adamant that Robyn was brain-dead. When the doctor entered the room, Robyn was singing, "He is the Lamb of God." I could tell it affected her by the emotion in her voice when she asked, "Is it OK that I follow Robyn's case?" I was glad to have her witness the miracle God performed in Robyn's life.

We spent five months at Primary Children's Hospital. When Robyn was discharged in February of 2008, she went home with a wheelchair; I told her that it was temporary too. The day I took Robyn home, I had no idea what I was getting into, but I knew that it was time for us both to go home. I also felt that if Robyn was going to get better, it would be with the love of family and friends supporting her.

During the time the medical team was discussing her release with us, a facility outside of Salt Lake City was suggested as a place for Robyn. My sister and I visited the facility. I was not impressed. When my sister and I walked out of the facility, we looked at each other and simultaneously said, "the devil is a lie."

When Robyn left home near midnight on October 4, 2007, we had no idea what was transpiring. I expected to return home with Robyn later the next morning. I certainly never anticipated being gone five months and returning with her disabled. We had no idea what to expect when we returned home in February of 2008.

Robyn was now in a wheelchair. She needed total assistance with personal care. She could not get in and out of a bathtub. She could not stand without assistance. I had to transfer her from the wheelchair to the bed, the couch, or a chair. The one thing she started to do was hold her fork better. We returned home to a new normal, one we would have to carve out for ourselves in a world totally unfamiliar to us.

——— ✧ ———

Robyn Oneida Edwards is my only daughter. I remember when I found out that I was pregnant, I prayed that God would allow me to have a little girl. When we did the sonogram and I received the news, I was overjoyed. I started buying bows and ribbons before she arrived. When she was a few months old, I would buy dresses, try them on her, and then prop her up on pillows in the bed, on the couch, and on her stuffed animals, while I took lots of photos. She was my little princess.

Okay, I realize this sounds crazy, but it was almost like going back twenty years to when I would make clothes for my dolls and have my dolls model them. My Mom, did not appreciate my creativeness as a child, probably because I once cut up one of her fur coats. Well, I just figured if she had a fur coat, my doll should have one too.

Dainty bows and barrettes did not last long. Robyn did not like the girly stuff I dressed her in. Well, I enjoyed my moments. When she was about nine or ten, I gave in a little and allowed her to select a portion of her clothes with my guidance of course. I would only force an outfit or two that I thought she just had to have. What can I say, I am a mother?

Like any mother, I have high hopes and dreams for my children. That has not changed. With all three of my children, when I found out I was pregnant my prayer was "Lord help me to raise this child in your ways." As he/she grows, "Lord help me to support them so that they will recognize all that they are in you."

Having had a Christian mother, I sometimes laugh at myself, because I know the thoughts I had of my own mom, so I can only imagine what my kids think of me. Well, I do not have to imagine because they often express their thoughts. Every now and then we have meetings where they are allowed to tell me things without reprisal. We often end the meetings laughing at each other and the naïve things they have done. Oh, no, I am not naïve; I know that they do not tell me everything. My hopes are that they realize that there is nothing too bad to share with me.

Robyn, like her brothers, had multiple talents. She loved music and could tap out songs on the piano by hearing them. So, I put her in piano classes. She did not appreciate my interest in her music abilities. I think this was one of the only times that she and I disagreed and I made her go anyway.

Robyn also loved to dance. I often received feedback after she and her older brother attended dances. I was often told they were the hit or main attraction. Ok, so, I am telling on myself, but once a friend and I went in through the backdoor entrance of a school dance. I was trying to get a sneak view of Robyn because I know my child. I wanted to see what she was doing. Robyn and her friends were always talking about the dance "the Stanky Leg." I wanted to see what it looked like. No, my efforts were in vain. The only thing I could see was a crowd of kids around someone. I imagined it could have been Robyn and her friends doing "the Stanky Leg." It was probably good that I never saw it.

At home, Robyn loved to cook. On Saturday mornings, she often cooked my favorite, bacon, egg and cheese omelet. She also cooked dinner some nights. I believe she thought she was a better cook than me. So, I let her do her thing. She also helped around the house and watched out for her younger brother. They were closer in age and were at the same school for a while.

She also enjoyed pulling pranks on her brothers. When her younger brother was about the second grade, she kissed him on his cheek at school because she said she was proud of him. It embarrassed him in front of his classmates. She then put her fist up at the kids around him just in case they made fun of him. After that incident, I think her younger brother avoided making contact with her at school.

Basketball was also a favorite of Robyn's. She enjoyed attending her older brother's games. When the referees called what she considered a bad foul against her brother's team, she yelled, "Open your eyes Ref." I often warned her that she was going to get us all thrown out of the gym. Needless to say, she has always thought highly of her older brother and adores him, which is usually aggravating to him. She calls him "Big Brah Brah."

During Robyn's seventh grade year she tried out for basketball. In previous years, she played in the YMCA basketball league. She reminded me a lot of her older brother. The long legs and arms that they struggled to coordinate but I figured, like her brother, she would soon gain control over her long limbs and become a good athlete, if that was what she chooses to do. During the weeks of the tryouts, she worked hard. We went to practice at the YMCA in the evenings after school and on the weekends. She really wanted to play on the team.

She was excited to get back to the school the evening that the coach was posting the list of students who made the team. We entered the school and headed towards the gym where everyone congregated. The coach appeared through the doors of the opposite hallway and posted the list of students who made the team. The kids took off in that direction. I saw Robyn look at the list, drop her head, look at me, and shake her head from side to side, as the tears began to roll down her cheeks. Before I made it to her, a friend who had a daughter try out too, tried to console her.

I wept for her on the inside. I grabbed her and hugged her and told her that it was OK. It was not over.

"You can still play for the YMCA," I said, as we walked to the car.

"Mom, that's not the same."

"Well, playing with them can increase your skills."

"That's not gonna help."

"Well, why don't we look into basketball camps?"

"OK," she said wiping the tears away.

I think the most challenging part of motherhood, for me, has been helping my children through their disappointments. It is difficult because it hurts me almost as much as it hurts them. As a parent you want to make it right, but how do you do that? Well, I realize sometimes I cannot make it right. I have to teach them that sometimes unfortunate things happen, but they decide how the situation manifests in their lives.

In Robyn's case, I encouraged her to fight for what she wanted. I told her if she wanted to play basketball, she had to work on her skills and try out again the following year. I think it helped until one of the kids who made the team called her a loser. At that point, I had to go back into my damage control mode again and redirect her.

Robyn decided to participate in the YMCA basketball league in the fall of her seventh-grade year. I was glad. She played hard and practiced hard. In the spring of 2007, she ran track. When she started running, she stopped drinking pops and eating junk food. She kept a count of her water intake. She exercised and stretched. I went to the track field with her to time her on her runs.

Her seventh-grade year she was one of the fastest runners on her track team, often running anchor position on the relay team. She was awesome. She ran the 100, 200 and a relay in which she was the anchor. I loved watching her.

"Go Robyn," I yelled as she began at the sound of the gun.

"C'mon Robyn." I could see her at the turn, coming up on the person to her left. Robyn was in the outside lane. "C'mon, C'mon, you can do it!" as she passed the person.

"Go! Robyn! Go! I yelled."

"Yea! She made it in first." I jumped up and down and hugged the person next to me. "She did it." I could see someone running out to her. The attendants lined them up in the place they came in. I settled back down on the bleacher.

"Mama, did you see me?" she asked.

"You didn't hear me screaming for you?" I asked. She shook her head from side to side and smiled. She hugged me and proceeded to the bleachers above, where her teammates were all seated. I was the proud mom, grinning from ear to ear.

——— ✧ ———

Robyn's stroke forever changed the trajectory of my family's future. I was no longer able to take my younger son to his basketball and soccer events, and I could not afford piano. I also missed my older son's basketball games and many senior events at school. We had to move from our house into an apartment.

The spring before Robyn's stroke she was inducted into the honor society. She was so excited about starting her eighth-grade year. She was enrolled in honors classes and was about to try out for basketball. I was even told by other players that the coach was looking for her to try out and asked about her. She was also on the track team. She had hopes of attending Yale University and one day running in the Olympics. All of her dreams were destroyed when Dr. Garland prescribed a drug that was the wrong drug even for his misdiagnosis of a rare migraine.

When Robyn returned to school in the spring of her eighth grade year, I became her scribe for her homework and she had an aide in school to scribe for her there. She was in a wheelchair and was still weak from the stroke. She only attended half the school day. She still needed a lot of assistance with her personal care. Although she missed five months of her eighth-grade year, because she was an honor student and had completed the necessary requirements, she was promoted to ninth grade.

When Robyn entered ninth grade during the 2009-2010 school year, she was still attending half the school day. The stroke affected her short-term memory and her processing. Consequently, she was no longer able to continue with the honors program. While she was no longer able to continue in honors classes, it was a blessing to be able to attend school, so she pressed forward. She still needed an aide to assist her in class, and I still scribed for her at home.

In January of 2009, I requested Robyn's rehabilitation doctor at Primary Children's Hospital (PCH) evaluate her for another stay of intense rehabilitation to assist with her walking. Robyn's physical therapist in Idaho Falls, had her in water therapy. She was now taking steps with her left leg, but she needed help stabilizing herself. The insurance approved a one month stay at PCH. My mom traveled to Idaho and stayed with my boys. Robyn and I spent a month at PCH in January of 2009.

—— ✧ ——

When we returned to Idaho Falls, Robyn was taking steps without assistance. My mom stayed an additional three months. Whenever my Mom left, I always felt a sinking feeling in my stomach. I think it was the reassurance her presence gave me.

Near the end of Robyn's ninth grade year, her track coach and the track team at Eagle Rock Jr. High School honored her at an assembly. I was contacted prior to the event, but Robyn was not aware of it. Because Robyn was still in her wheelchair at school, no one was aware that she was walking without assistance. When the coach called her out to the gym floor to accept an honorary track uniform, she rose from her wheelchair and walked out to accept it. It was a tearful, exciting moment for everyone, especially her teammates.

When Robyn entered her tenth-grade year she planned to attend the entire day. Members of the IEP team were not sure she would be able to endure the entire day and neither was I. Plans were not in place for her to attend all day. Robyn's aide from Eagle Rock Jr. High continued with her in high school. The aide was also not aware that Robyn would attend full time in tenth grade. For that reason, Robyn was assigned an additional aide for the afternoon session.

Robyn had a couple of incidents. She has left-side neglect in her left eye. As a result, she does not see in her left peripheral vision, so she occasionally walks into people and things. One day she walked into a pole at school and got a nice lump on her head to remind her to look left when she walked around school.

Even though Robyn was walking more, her doctors and therapists were not sure she could endure an entire day of walking from class to class. A prescription for a motorized wheelchair was ordered. By the time the necessary assessments were completed for approval of the chair, Robyn was walking through the hallways of Skyline High School without assistance. The motorized chair was not ordered.

While Robyn's junior high years after the stroke were challenging, they were not as challenging as her high school years. Robyn and I were plummeted into the world of special education by the damage to her brain from the stroke, but my expectations regarding her education had not changed. What I found in Robyn's case and common in many schools attempting to educate Traumatic Brain Injury (TBI) students, is that most schools are not equipped to meet the needs of a child with a TBI. While Individualized Education Plans (IEP) are supposed to be tailored to the needs of the student, the specific needs of a child with TBI can be overwhelming for all involved in planning. Many TBI students still have the ability to learn, but it takes a lot more time and effort on the part of educators. Usually more than the average school program has allotted, which creates a struggle for the administrators, teachers and parents. I found this to be true for us too.

During Robyn's tenth grade year, she started complaining about her aide. This was the same aide she had when she returned to school in 2008. I listened and thought that it was more of an age difference than anything. Her aide and I were close in age. I was comfortable with the aide. She helped Robyn to adjust when she returned to school and was very helpful to me, but Robyn had a problem with her. I initially asked Robyn to consider whether it was the aide or just the inconvenience of having someone with her all day at school. If it was inconvenience, it was something she had to endure because she needed the assistance of an aide.

Near the end of Robyn's first semester of her tenth-grade year, she started making comments about how she hated school. This was new because regardless of her struggles, school was always a highlight. I thought it was the lack of continuity in having two aides. I mentioned this to the case manager on the IEP team.

The afternoon aide was a young girl. Robyn complained about the afternoon aid assisting others when she needed assistance. When I picked Robyn up from school, I sometimes found Robyn sitting at a table and the younger aide reading a book.

One day Robyn came home from school and it was obvious that something was wrong. When I inquired about her gloomy mood, she said the younger aide did not like her. I suggested that maybe she was reading too much into the young lady's actions. Robyn went on to tell me what happened during that day. Robyn was using the bathroom and had trouble getting the tissue off the roll. She requested the young lady's assistance. The aide entered the stall huffing and puffing, offending Robyn. Robyn said the aide often made her feel bad about asking for assistance.

It is difficult for any person with a disability, especially those who have been independent, to ask for help regarding their personal needs. For the aide of a disabled person to degrade and take away the dignity of the disabled person, by making their request for help appear disgusting or offensive, is unacceptable. I called a meeting with the IEP team and asked for her to be removed. I think it took a letter to the school district office before any action was taken.

The aid situation was not totally resolved. Robyn still had the older aid she complained about before the younger aid came aboard. I thought Robyn was being too hard on the older lady. The older aid had been with Robyn since she returned to school her eighth grade year. She had also been a big help to me with keeping up on homework assignments. While Robyn continually complained about the older lady, she never gave me anything concrete.

After the younger aide was removed, the other aide was brought on full-time. As the second semester began, I noticed in the daily logs that Robyn seemed to regress, and I questioned the comments of the aide. I also started asking more questions and paying more attention to Robyn's comments regarding the aide. I finally asked for the aide to be replaced because it appeared that the two were having problems communicating, and this I knew was affecting Robyn's learning. My request was met with opposition from some of the IEP team members.

I had also started visiting the school more, especially during testing, because with Robyn's short term memory loss she needed prompting. Her aide did not appear to know how to assist her in this area. At one point my integrity was challenged while I assisted Robyn with a test. I called a meeting with the IEP team. During the meeting, I informed them that I needed help; if they had a problem with the way I prompted Robyn, then help me find a better method. Instead of finding problems, help me find a solution. The teacher of the class in which Robyn tested, started testing Robyn herself. This was very helpful to Robyn, and I was thankful to God.

After that was resolved, one day the aide wrote me a long note in the daily log stating what Robyn was not able to do and the enormous amount of work Robyn was behind on. She gave me a long list of what she had to do for Robyn because Robyn either would not or could not do it herself. Some of the things she listed, Robyn had been doing at home for a while. I wondered why Robyn was not performing at school.

At this point, I was starting to believe that Robyn's complaints about this aide were valid. My response to the aides list was not very nice. I informed the aide that I did not want her working with Robyn, ever again. I followed that note with a letter to the principal and the district office. I later apologized to the aide because it was not my intent to offend her, but I wanted her removed as Robyn's aide.

I appreciated the assistance that the older aide gave Robyn, especially helping re-acclimate Robyn to the school environment. What I refused to accept was the school administration's resistance to change directions when it was needed. It was very frustrating, but I am thankful that I had some members on the IEP team that understood the necessity for change and that it was not personal. It was necessary for Robyn's healing and growth.

The IEP representative from the district office helped find another aide for Robyn. She too was an older lady, and Robyn did not like her. With this aide Robyn's complaints were different. This aide drilled Robyn. When I picked Robyn up from school Robyn's books were still open and they were still studying. Robyn said she was overbearing. I told Robyn we were not going to find the perfect aide but with this aide, regardless of her faults, she appeared to want Robyn to succeed.

One of the highlights of Robyn's tenth grade year, was when one of the counselors of Eagle Rock Jr. High School asked her to be the keynote speaker at their Honor Society Induction Ceremony the spring of 2010. Robyn's younger brother was also being inducted into the Honors Society. I felt blessed that he was able to maintain his focus throughout all we endured. As a parent it was an honor to have him inducted and have Robyn address the young people and encourage them to never give up. At the end of Robyn's speech, she read one of her favorite poems by DR. W. Hubert Brewster, “I'm Determined to Be Somebody Someday.”

Robyn also joined Skyline High School's choir. She also attended other school events and continued to cheer on the Grizzlies football teams. She continued to push forward and enjoyed her classes and her teachers.

In Robyn's eleventh grade year, I attended Geometry class with her as her aide because it was difficult for me to understand the aide’s notes and Robyn was not able to recall and explain them. Because Robyn's short-term memory was affected by the stroke, it took her longer to remember information and to process it.

In the spring of 2011, Robyn decided to go out for track again. Of course, I was astonished when one of the coaches of Skyline approached me and informed me that Robyn needed to be cleared by her doctor to try out. I took Robyn to her primary care doctor, and he thought it would be a good challenge for her. Robyn began meeting after school for track practice. The coaches assured me not to worry. They allowed her to go as far as she could with it, but it interfered with her occupational and speech therapy in the afternoon, so she had to quit.

In the fall of 2011, Robyn and her younger brother, tried out for the musical play "Hair Spray." They both were cast in the ensemble. I was proud of them both. It took a lot of determination and boldness on Robyn's part. It also took a lot of tolerance on her brother's part. I was also thankful for the directors and the compassion of everyone involved for being inclusive.

Robyn also decided to run for female activity director of her senior class for the 2011-2012 school year. One day while picking Robyn up from school, I was approached by one of Robyn's teachers. They were concerned that with Robyn's popularity among her senior class, she might be elected female activity director. They did not think she would be able to meet the demands of the position. They suggested creating an assistant activity director position for her if she won. I never asked how the election turned out. Robyn was the assistant female activity director of her senior class of 2011-2012. She was ecstatic and I was excited for her.

By Robyn's twelfth grade year, I was glad that we were through with math classes. Eleventh grade geometry had taken a toll on me. The year started as usual, with an IEP meeting in which we established goals for the year. Robyn was excited and was ready to get started. I allowed her to attend events without me. Her classmates picked her up for the games and brought her home.

I returned to work in March of 2011. With Robyn and her younger brother's activities I was overwhelmed, but thankful. My younger son played violin in the school orchestra, and he started taking piano lessons again. He also started taking Karate lessons from our pastor at New Hope Church of God in Christ. My younger son sacrificed so much after Robyn returned home; I was excited to get him back into activities.

My older son left for college in the fall of 2009, so a lot of responsibilities fell on my younger son. Most of his extracurricular activities ended when his older brother left for college. My younger son cooked and cleaned after school while I took Robyn to physical, occupational, and speech therapy. After returning home from therapy, I assisted her with homework which usually took the remainder of the evening.

During Robyn's senior year, she started taking Rolling Shuttle to therapy session. Rolling Shuttle is a transportation service in the Idaho Falls area for the disabled. This helped a lot and allowed me to enroll my younger son into piano again and take him to his lessons.

Chapter 3

Dr. Erich Garland & Idaho Board of Medicine

You pushed me violently, that I might fall. But the Lord helped me. The Lord is my strength and song, and he has become my salvation

Psalms 118:13-14 (NKJV).

On September 14, 2013, I made myself stop and check the mailbox. Checking the mail is probably one of the most dreaded on my list of tasks, since taking on Robyn's medical malpractice lawsuit. For this reason, I had not checked it in seven days, and the box was overflowing. As I scanned through the pile of mail, I saw the letter from Idaho Board of Medicine. I pulled it out and started to open it, but my kids were impatient. "Mom, can't you do that at the house." I placed the letter at the top of the stack. By now, my heartbeat started to increase.

I dropped Robyn and her brother off near the staircase on the side of the apartment and I headed to the garage. As I backed the SUV into the garage, I had to stop and correct several times. It was now difficult to concentrate on what I was doing. This is why I hated checking the mail. Usually, I had my son check it and hold it until we made it to the apartment. I took a deep breath, calmed down, and backed the SUV into the narrow opening.

After I made it into the apartment, I placed the mail on the dining room table with the letter from Idaho Board of Medicine on top. I wondered why I was receiving another letter so soon. I received a letter dated August 21, 2013, that stated the board staff had received the complaint and would update us on the status of the complaint every 45-60 days because their investigation could take months.

Prior to receiving the letter from the board of medicine, I received a call from the Idaho Falls Police department on August 19, 2013. Last year when I attempted to file a police report against Dr. Garland and Robyn's Malpractice Attorneys for using fraudulent documents to intimidate me, they refused to take a report. Finally, a report was taken on July 31, 2013. Officer Barnes was the officer assigned to investigate.

Apparently, Dr. Garland wrote a letter October 1, 2007 which, according to Officer Barnes, led the Bonneville County Prosecutor to consider discontinuing the investigation. The letter contains the same fabrications in the deposition regarding Robyn having migraine headaches. He even added a lot of information that we did not give him. Robyn made the local news that year and there were several articles about her in the paper and on TV. I imagine this is where he obtained a lot of information about her. He also mentioned in the letter the MRI which I requested on October 2, 2007. In addition, he notated the date of the MRI which was confirmed on October 3, 2007. I asked Officer Barnes if he had thoroughly examined the letter. He said he had.

"Officer Barnes, how can a letter written on October 1, 2007, contain information of events that occurred on the 2nd and 3rd of October? If you check the files, the MRI that Garland mentions in the letter was requested by me on October 2nd and the MRI was confirmed on the 3rd. How could Dr. Garland include this information in a letter he signed and dated October 1, 2007?" I asked.

"Well, I went through the records, and I don't recall seeing that information," Officer Barnes replied.

"Did you request medical records from Dr. Garland? Because if you did, this information is in the files. Officer Barnes, I know what's in the files because I have copies. I don't see how you can investigate without this information."

"I have looked through the records and I don't have this information. Will you send me the information?"

"Yes, I will email you the information."

When the call ended, I thought about others who could possibly verify that the MRI was not ordered until Tuesday, October 2, 2007. I emailed Officer Barnes:

Officer Barnes,
While I was searching through my files, I thought about two witnesses that I spoke with the evening of October 1st, 2007. I spoke with Robyn's father, XXX, who is a registered nurse and my sister, XXX, who is also a registered nurse and they both questioned why an MRI was not ordered.

I copied them on this letter because they encouraged me to get one ordered. You can get information from either of them because I was in contact with them both.

I am sure both of them would be willing to talk to you.

Sincerely,

Veverly Edwards

The police attempts to deceive me are incredulous. The letter the police referenced was purportedly written by Dr. Garland on October 1, 2007. Here lies the problem, how can he predict me calling back on October 2, 2007 to request the MRI? How would he know the date of the MRI, and record it in a letter he wrote on October 1, 2007? If the letter proves anything, it is Dr. Garland's attempts to deceive.

Robyn had an afternoon appointment with Dr. Garland on that day. He diagnosed her with a rare form of migraine that caused numbing sensations and prescribed two drugs: Zomig and Depracote. I questioned Garland because I had a sister who had migraine headaches as a child. I was not aware of a migraine that caused numbness in the limbs, and Robyn did not have headaches. He assured me that this was the case and added that she would probably grow out of it. He also stated that she may develop headaches at some point and that I could also give her ibuprofen. When I asked him to order an MRI, he refused because he did not recommend it. In the letter he makes it appear that he and I consulted and agreed to order it. The letter follows this page.

IDAHO FALLS NEUROLOGY

Erich W. Garland, M.D.
Board Certified

October 1, 2007

Ron W. Porter, M.D.
2375 Coronado Street
Idaho Falls, ID 83404

Re: Robin Edwards

Dear Dr. Porter:

I had the pleasure to see and examine Robin Edwards in my office on October 1, 2007. She is a 13 year old African-American who presents at your request concerning transient episodes of numbness in her hands, lower legs, and face. This has occurred on several occasions the past two months. She may get a sense of disequilibrium. Episodes can be brief, five to ten minutes in duration, sometimes less. A headache will usually occur after a spell. She has no associated visual distortions. She may develop fatigue. Headache pain can last hours or sometimes the entire day. These episodes may occur more than once a day. Nausea occurs occasionally but is not disabling. Her mother reports that she had a spell in my office after arriving for her appointment and now has a headache.

Past Medical History: Remarkable only for knee arthroscopic surgery. She has not been previously diagnosed with migraines. She has no history of sickle cell disease.

Allergies to Medications: None.

Medications Used: None.

Family History: Remarkable for asthma, numbness, hypertension, depression and multiple sclerosis.

Social History: She is currently in the 8th grade. She plays basketball and track and is very good at it. She is not using caffeine. She has no problems with sleep.

3920 Washington Parkway, Idaho Falls, Idaho 83404
(208) 227-0158 Fax: (208) 227-0159

Garland 00034

Ron W. Porter, M.D.
October 1, 2007
Page 2

Re: Robin Edwards

Review of Systems: Overall her health has been good. She has dizziness, numbness, weakness, problems with balance and sometimes expressive difficulties when headaches are present. Otherwise review of fourteen systems is unremarkable except as described above.

Physical Examination: She is alert and appears in no obvious discomfort or distress. She is oriented to place, time and situation and demonstrates appropriate short-term memory, attention and cognition. Blood pressure is 120/70, heart rate 70 and regular, respirations 16. Ear, nose and throat exams are normal. The neck is supple. The lungs are clear in all fields. Cardiac exam demonstrates regular rate and rhythm without murmurs or gallops. Skin and extremity exams are normal to inspection. She has no rashes or edema. The nail beds are normal. She has no skeletal deformities. Neurologic assessment: Fundi and disks are normal. Extraocular movements are intact in all fields of gaze. She has no nystagmus. Pupils are 3 mm equal and reactive to light. Facial sensation is normal. Facial muscle strength is normal. Sternocleidomastoid and trapezius muscles are strong. Tongue demonstrates normal movement. Motor exam demonstrates normal strength and muscle tone in the upper and lower limbs. Deep tendon reflexes are 2+/2 symmetric. Babinski stimulation produces a bilateral flexor response. Sensory exam demonstrates normal pin, temperature, touch, vibration and proprioception. There is no asymmetry on sensory exam. Gait, balance and postural reflexes are normal. Cerebellar exam is normal.

Impression: Classical migraine by history. No history of sleep impairment. She has a normal neurologic exam.

We will begin a trial with Depakote 250 mg at bedtime. I have provided the mother and patient educational materials concerning migraine and samples of Zomig 5 mg ZMT to take with early onset of a spell. Because of some unusual features of her headache, we will get an MRI of the brain. This is scheduled at Teton Radiology for October 9, 2007 at 3:30 p.m.

I have asked her to follow up in six weeks. She has been instructed to call my office if she has any problems in the meantime.

Garland 00035

Ron W. Porter, M.D.
October 1, 2007
Page 3

Re: Robin Edwards

Sincerely,

Erich W. Garland, M.D.

EWG/MT42

Dictated not read.

could determine who actually made the entries on the documents.

Also, when we asked about Mr. Mason's findings Mr. Nalder and Mr. Barton discounted his abilities and findings and stated that he didn't have the experience that they had.

4. *I do not believe I should pay Mr. Nalder anything because he has attempted to undermine this case and help the opposing side by attempting to intimidate me.*

5. *My ex-husband dismissed his interests based on the lies that Mr. Nalder told regarding the expert witness and my testimony. Yet, a letter existed before we even met that shows Mr. XXX had not recanted and still held to the same statement. Mr. Nalder has presented false information to intimidate us to dismiss this case.*

6. *My desire is to file felony charges of fraud and falsification against Mr. Nalder and Mr. Barton.*

I was under a lot of duress when I filed the first complaint with the bar. I also had no idea the extent to which Mr. Nalder had undermined me. When the Board sent me a letter in December of 2012, stating they found no grounds for my complaint, I was disappointed but not discouraged. The Idaho Bar's letter is on the next page.

ISB
IDAHO STATE BAR

Office of Bar Counsel
525 West Jefferson • P. O. Box 895 • Boise, Idaho 83701
(208) 334-4500 • Fax: (208) 334-2764
www.idaho.gov/isb

December 14, 2012

PERSONAL & CONFIDENTIAL

Veverly M. Edwards
555 S. Old Butte Hwy, #602
Idaho Falls, ID 83402

Re: Grievance against G. Lance Nalder
ISB File No. 12-C187G

Dear Ms. Edwards:

This responds to your complaint to the Idaho State Bar against attorney G. Lance Nalder.

It is my responsibility as Deputy Bar Counsel for the Idaho State Bar to review each complaint in light of the Idaho Bar Commission Rules and the Idaho Rules of Professional Conduct. The standard of proof in attorney discipline matters is clear and convincing evidence. Clear and convincing evidence is a high standard of proof requiring substantial corroboration to establish facts otherwise disputed.

We have reviewed your complaint and the materials submitted with your complaint. We recognize that you believe Mr. Nalder violated the Idaho Rules of Professional Conduct. However, pursuant to Idaho Bar Commission Rule 504(b)(1) and based upon our initial review, we have determined that there is not clear and convincing evidence that this matter is founded or within the purview of the Idaho Rules of Professional Conduct ("I.R.P.C.").

The material facts follow. Between April 2009 and May 30, 2012, Mr. Nalder and co-counsel, Breck Barton, jointly represented you, your teenage daughter, Robyn Edwards ("Robyn"), and your ex-husband, [redacted], in a medical malpractice case, *Robyn Edwards et al., v. Erich Garland, M.D.*, Bonneville County Case No. CV 2010-3994. Dr. Garland was represented by attorney Terrence Jones.

Dr. Garland is a neurologist. In October 2007, Dr. Garland diagnosed Robyn, who was 13-years-old at that time, as suffering from migraine headaches. He prescribed Zomig, a migraine headache medicine. You have informed us that Robyn has a rare condition called Moyamoya which Dr. Garland failed to diagnose. After taking the medicine prescribed by Dr. Garland for several days, Robyn had a severe stroke which left her permanently disabled.

In April 2009, you and Mr. Edwards retained Mr. Nalder to prosecute a medical malpractice claim against Dr. Garland. You signed a 40% contingency fee contract. In July 2010, Mr. Nalder filed the lawsuit, *Robyn Edwards et al., v. Erich Garland, M.D*, asserting that Dr. Garland's treatment of Robyn fell below the standard of care in Idaho and claiming

Veverly M. Edwards
Page 2
December 14, 2012

damages on behalf of Robyn related to the treatment, and on behalf of you and Mr. Edwards as her natural parents.

Dr. Garland contested the claims. Between July 2010 and April 2012, the case was litigated. The Court denied Dr. Garland's Motion for Summary Judgment, discovery was exchanged and depositions were conducted. Meanwhile, Mr. Nalder retained an expert medical witness, Dr. [redacted] M.D., who reviewed all of the medical records, discovery and depositions. In March 2012, Dr. [redacted] wrote a letter in which he noted inconsistencies in some of the statements and records, but essentially concluded that the Zomig was a substantial contributing factor to Robyn's stroke and Dr. Garland had breached the applicable standard of care by prescribing it to her. Dr. Garland also had retained his own expert medical witnesses, who concluded that based on the totality of circumstances, Dr. Garland had not breached the standard of care in Idaho because Moyamoya was such a rare disorder. A jury trial was scheduled for October 23, 2012.

In April 2012, Mr. Nalder and Mr. Barton informed you and Mr. Edwards that pursuant to the terms of the contingency fee contract which permitted their withdrawal, they were discontinuing their involvement in the case. In summary, Mr. Nalder informed you that in recent telephone conversations, Dr. [redacted] had retreated from his previous position that Dr. Garland had breached the standard of care for failing to diagnose that Robyn had the rare disorder Moyamoya. Mr. Nalder informed you that he did not believe that it could be proven that the ingestion of Zomig was the cause of Robyn's stroke. Mr. Nalder also informed you that he had concerns that your testimony was inconsistent with some of the evidence as to Robyn's symptoms at the time she was examined by Dr. Garland.

On May 4, 2012, Mr. Edwards voluntarily dismissed himself from the lawsuit. You objected to Mr. Nalder's withdrawal. Consequently, Mr. Nalder and Mr. Barton filed a Motion to Withdraw with the Court requesting permission to withdraw from yours and Robyn's representation. That motion was granted after a hearing on May 14, 2012. You continued to represent yourself *pro se* until October 18, 2012, when you dismissed the lawsuit.

You are dissatisfied that Mr. Nalder withdrew from the representation. You suspect that Mr. Nalder cooperated with opposing counsel to create inconsistent paperwork and medical records that were provided by Dr. Garland in discovery. You argue that Mr. Nalder may have helped create a forged patient intake form and extensive examination notes and medical records that allegedly did not exist prior to the litigation. You allege that Mr. Nalder has failed to provide you with anything in writing from Dr. [redacted] that substantiates that the expert had changed his opinion about whether Dr. Garland violated the standard of care. Finally, you contend that Mr. Nalder failed to pursue your objectives in the representation and engaged in a possible criminal conspiracy to falsify evidence and sabotage the case. You have refused to pay any of his costs.

39

Veverly M. Edwards
Page 3
December 14, 2012

You contend that Mr. Nalder violated I.R.P.C. 1.2 and 1.16(d) or that those rules are implicated. I.R.P.C. 1.2(a) provides that a lawyer shall abide by a client's decisions concerning the objectives of representation, and as required by Rule 1.4, shall consult with the client as to the means by which they are to be pursued. A lawyer shall abide by a client's decision whether to settle a matter. I.R.P.C. 1.16(d) provides that upon termination of representation, a lawyer shall take steps to the extent reasonably practicable to protect a client's interests, such as giving reasonable notice to the client, allowing time for employment of other counsel, surrendering papers and property to which the client is entitled and refunding any advance payment of fee or expense that has not been earned or incurred. Based on our investigation and the materials we reviewed, we do not find clear and convincing evidence that your contention that Mr. Nalder violated I.R.P.C. 1.2 and 1.16(d) is founded.

Comment 2 to I.R.P.C. 1.2 states in pertinent part:

> Clients normally defer to the special knowledge and skill of their lawyer with respect to the means to be used to accomplish their objectives, particularly with respect to technical, legal and tactical matters.

A lawyer therefore has independent professional discretion to decide the means to accomplish a client's objectives after consultation with the client, particularly with respect to decisions involving legal judgment and tactics. Moreover, Mr. Nalder's obligations to pursue your objectives under I.R.P.C. 1.2 are tempered by his obligations under other rules to render candid advice and to bring meritorious proceedings.

In his letter dated April 13, 2012, Mr. Nalder informed you that he had substantial doubts that your medical malpractice claim was viable and he explained the specific reasons why. Mr. Nalder provided you with reasonable notice that he intended to withdraw, and he described your options and the steps he was willing to take to protect your interests upon withdrawal. We recognize that you believe that you had an extremely strong malpractice case against Dr. Garland and we appreciate that you are suspicious of, and disagree with, Mr. Nalder's assessment of its prospects and decision to withdraw. However, we do not find credible clear and convincing evidence that Mr. Nalder unethically cooperated with opposing counsel, committed fraud, or otherwise failed to abide by your decisions concerning the objectives of representation. We also do not find clear and convincing evidence that upon termination of representation, Mr. Nalder failed to take steps to the extent reasonably practicable to protect your interests. We therefore do not find clear and convincing evidence that your contention that Mr. Nalder violated I.R.P.C. 1.2 and 1.16(d) is founded.

Consequently, we do not find clear and convincing evidence that your grievance is founded or to support a continuation of this investigation. Pursuant to Idaho Bar Commission Rule 509(b)(1), we will therefore discontinue the investigation and proceedings concerning this matter and close our file because it is unfounded or beyond the purview of

Veverly M. Edwards
Page 4
December 14, 2012

the Idaho Rules of Professional Conduct and we do not find clear and convincing evidence of any violation of the Rules.

You may seek review of this Bar Counsel disposition by filing a written request for such review, stating the reasons for the request, with the Clerk of the Professional Conduct Board, Idaho State Bar, P.O. Box 895, Boise, Idaho 83701, within fourteen (14) days of receipt of this disposition. The Clerk shall send a copy of the request for review to the Respondent.

Thereafter, consistent with Idaho Bar Commission Rule 509, the Chair of the Professional Conduct Board will appoint a Hearing Committee to review the matter. Within fourteen (14) days of the assignment to a Hearing Committee, the Clerk will notify the Grievant, Respondent and Bar Counsel of the assignment. The Clerk will forward a copy of the request for review, together with the file concerning the matter, to the Hearing Committee, Grievant, and the Respondent. Consistent with Rule 509, the Hearing Committee will review the matter upon the record before it, unless either party requests a hearing. If the party seeking review of this disposition desires such a hearing, he or she shall so state in the request for review. If the other party desires a hearing, he or she shall make a request, in writing, to the Clerk of the Professional Conduct Board at the address listed above, within seven (7) days of being served with the request for review.

The Hearing Committee will review the existing record prior to holding a hearing, if one is requested. All hearings shall be by telephone, unless the Hearing Committee prescribes another method. If a hearing is held, the parties shall be permitted to file briefs and make oral argument related to the grievance under review, and the Hearing Committee may ask questions regarding the record before it. The Hearing Committee chair may limit the presentation at the hearing, in his or her sole discretion. All written materials related to the hearing shall be sent to the Clerk, who shall disseminate them to all parties and to the Hearing Committee.

For matters relating to the time for rendering the decision, service of the decision and the effect of the Hearing Committee decision, please see Idaho Bar Commission Rule 509. A copy of that rule is provided for your convenience.

Thank you for your consideration.

Sincerely,

Julia A. Crossland
Deputy Bar Counsel

JAC:agg
Enclosure

41

I had a couple of weeks to file for a hearing by a Professional Conduct Committee to review the case. I filed for the hearing. I had more information regarding Mr. Nalder's negligence and unethical behavior than when I first filed.

Not only had Mr. Nalder given misinformation regarding the facts of the case, but when I decided to continue with the case, in retaliation, he filed everyone's claim in the case, but mine. He filed a claim on behalf of Robyn, her father, and all the experts who had to be paid for their services. I was not made aware of this until much later. I figured this was just another of his schemes to make sure the case did not go any further.

I am sure that anyone who called Mr. Nalder regarding the case received the same lies he told my ex-husband and his attorney. Now, Mr. Nalder could also use the fact that my ex-husband dismissed with prejudice, making me look like a distraught mother in denial. I contacted many attorneys, some knew Mr. Barton and refused to take the case. This may be why he was brought on. It appears he was more reputable than Mr. Nalder.

I eventually had to file Pro Se to represent the case myself. Filing Pro Se allowed me to represent the case in both Robyn's and my interest. Since my finances were considerably challenged from Robyn's prom, graduation, and my older son's airfare home, I asked my older brother to buy a book for me. He purchased the book "How to Represent Yourself in Court" and sent it to me. I began my journey through the court processes of Bonneville County Civil Court and started filing motions.

I initially had no idea that Mr. Nalder did not file my claim in the case. When Robyn turned 18, June 24, 2012, she was considered an adult. About a month after her birthday, I received a motion from the defense attorney to have me removed from the case. Now that Robyn was an adult, I could not represent the case because I had no claim in it. I searched for an attorney to represent Robyn. We did not find one. Robyn filed Pro Se to represent herself. In October we filed to have it dismissed without prejudice meaning she could refile.

Months before Mr. Nalder's meeting in April, I forwarded my tax and financial information to him so that he could calculate my claim. The information I forwarded was in response to a letter he sent requesting my financial information so that he could file my claim in the case. Mr. Nalder's request was in response to a motion from Dr. Garland's attorney requesting all claims in the case. When I submitted my information to the assistant in his office working on Robyn's case, she informed me that my ex-husband had not turned in his tax information. I sent my ex-husband a text to let him know that they were waiting on his information. So, I found it interesting that Mr. Nalder was able to submit my ex-husband's claim and not mine.

Mr. Nalder had issues with me early on, but I was too bogged down with other issues and discounted the difference in how he interacted with me and my ex-husband. During the deposition, when the opposing side asked if the parents' were filing a claim, Mr. Nalder stated only my ex-husband was. My ex-husband and I looked at each other and then at him. We stopped the deposition to update him that we were both filing a claim. When the deposition resumed, Mr. Nalder acknowledged my claim. His behavior towards me was questionable throughout the proceedings. A copy of the page of the deposition showing Mr. Nalder first denying my claim and later acknowledging my claim is on the following page. It starts on page 38 line 24.

Page 38

give you all of my education?
Q. I'm just interested in the years you attended and any degree you obtained.
A. Okay. So then I started at the University of Moscow in August of 2004. I completed that and my specialist degree in 2010. I actually finished my master's degree before Robyn got sick, but I didn't realize it, because she'd gotten sick that year.
Q. So you completed your bachelor's in communications from the University of Memphis in '87?
A. Yes.
Q. And then you started to work on your masters in 2004 and completed that in 2010?
A. I did.
Q. And who is the institution? Was it the University of Idaho?
A. It was.
Q. And that's a master's degree in what?
A. Secondary education.
Q. Okay. And do you have, as a result of any of your work or educational background, any education in medicine of any kind?
A. I don't.
Q. Are we seeking lost wages for either of the parents?

Page 39

MR. NALDER: Not for Veverly. I'll have to check with Robert. I don't believe so. But there was a period of time when they were not able to work. I guess the best answer is I'm not sure right now in light of the questions that you've asked. Let's take a break.
MR. JONES: Okay.
(Recess.)
MR. JONES: Back on the record.
MR. NALDER: Yes. The answer to your question is yes. I've spoken with Veverly and she was employed, I think, at two different jobs at the time of this incident. Robert advises that he was -- he had to take FMLA leave without pay subsequent to this incident. So, yes, we are making a lost wages claim.
MR. JONES: All right. With that I will proceed asking additional questions about your work background. You indicated that you completed your communications degree in 1987?
A. I did.
Q. Just walk us forward since then, what type of jobs you've had since then?
A. You want since what year? Give me the year you want.
Q. Since 1987 to the present.
A. I worked for Federal Express from 1985 to

Page 40

about 1993.
Q. What did you do for them?
A. '95 or '96, I'm sorry. Let's say '96.
Q. So you worked for Federal Express?
A. Yes. I worked in their --
MR. NALDER: Let him ask the question, Veverly. You're jumping the gun all the time and you have to stop that.
Q. (BY MR. JONES) It seems like if we're in a casual conversation it's quite normal for people to talk over one another, but with the court reporter here it changes to a more formal sort of approach. I ask the question, you answer the question. I'll let you have time to answer the question, but you need to let me ask the question.
So you worked for Federal Express from 1985 until 1996; is that correct?
A. Give me a moment. I'm thinking about the years. (Pause.) '87 to '96, yes.
Q. And what did you do for Federal Express?
A. I worked as a sorter for two years. I worked in customer care for about eight years. I went through their management program. I left there -- that's it for Federal Express.
Q. So you were a sorter and in customer care

Page 41

and then you said you had applied for something?
A. I went through their management program and was endorsed into that. I was able to apply for a management position.
Q. Did you have any management positions within Federal Express?
A. No.
Q. What was the reason you left Federal Express in 1996?
A. I left because of the responsibilities at home with the kids. I took a home position with Federal Express.
Q. What years did you have a home position with them?
A. That was a contract. It was actually -- approximately from February of '96 to about February of '97.
Q. What did you do for work after 1997?
A. Licensed real estate agent.
Q. And how long were you in that capacity?
A. About 10 years.
Q. When was the last time you sold anything with a real estate license?
A. I can't give you a month. The year was approximately 2006.

When I filed my second complaint, I added Mr. Nalder's failure to file my claim in the case. I found it difficult to believe that Mr. Nalder fulfilled his responsibilities to me as a client, without filing my interests in the case. How could he have met his obligation to me as my attorney, when he failed to file my claim in the case?

I also included my concern with Mr. Nalder filing a subpoena for copies of my EEO complaint because it was during an active investigation. My complaint against an employer for an EEO violation had nothing to do with the malpractice lawsuit. As a matter of fact, I had even discussed this with Ben Mason, the attorney in Mr. Nalder's Law Firm who initiated our complaint against Dr. Garland because it happened after the malpractice case was in progress. He did not see an issue.

So why would Mr. Nalder, who was supposedly representing me, draw the attention of the Human Rights Commission to the malpractice lawsuit? Why would he allow anyone to distract or potentially compromise the outcome of an EEO investigation? I am not sure what the laws are regarding someone filling a subpoena for copies of an EEO complaint during an active investigation, but certainly there should be stricter rules to protect the integrity of the EEO process and the interest of the person filing the complaint.

I also informed the Professional Conduct Committee about Mr. Nalder forwarding my personal information to my ex-husband. I noticed when Mr. Nalder sent me a copy of the EEO complaint, it appeared that a copy was also sent to my ex-husband. So I called Mr. Nalder's office and asked why they were forwarding my information to my ex-husband, it was apparent that we were divorced. The assistant replied that it was because he was a party to the lawsuit. I then asked, why I had not received any of my ex-husband's information. She was supposed to get back with me on that question, but she never did.

The following is the second complaint, and my request for a hearing before an Idaho Bar Professional Conduct Committee. I have taken out some identifiable information and placed XXX in its place.

January 13, 2013

Clerk of The Professional Conduct Board
Idaho State Bar
Boise, Idaho 83701

Re: Grievance against G. Lance Nalder
ISB FileNo. XXX

To Whom It May Concern:

I recently received the letter regarding the decision of the Idaho Bar Counsel (dated December 14, 2012), stating that they did not find clear and convincing evidence that my grievance was founded. I moved to California in August of 2012 and did not receive this letter until much later. I called your office and XXX informed me that she would give me until the middle of January to respond.

I am requesting a review/hearing because I do believe Lance Nalder's actions were negligent, unethical and blatant. I am even more convinced after reviewing the filings in these proceedings that his intent was to undermine the testimony of the Plaintiff Veverly Edwards in the Case of Edwards vs. Garland in which he represented all three Plaintiffs.

> 1) *Lance Nalder and Breck Barton did not initially represent this case. Benjamin Mason did. This is relevant because Lance Nalder was not informed/or was intentionally giving misinformation on what had transpired in this case. In the letter dated April, 13, 2012, in which he states his reasons for dismissal, on the third page-first paragraph he states, "While we believe that we can put together sufficient information to avoid the entry of a summary judgment against you (even though we expect that such a motion will be filed by Dr. Garland) we do not believe that you will prevail at the time of hearing."*
>
> *Consequently, a summary judgment had already been entered and denied by Judge Tingey on March 8, 2011. I am*

forwarding a copy of it. My point is Lance Nalder either was lying or had no clue of the proceedings in this case. I had never heard of Breck Barton until the meeting on April 11, 2012. Lane Blake had been handling everything. Even when Nalder supposedly prepped me for the deposition, his idea of prepping me was to tell me he hoped I remembered everything.

2) Benjamin Mason was first to recognize the inconsistency in Dr. Garland's records. I am forwarding emails that my ex-husband forwarded to me from Ben Mason discussing the inconsistencies during his deposition of Dr. Garland. The email was sent from Mason on January 12, 2011.

I assure you my concerns are not unfounded. If Lance Nalder had not shown me the false records in an attempt to intimidate me on April 11, 2012, I would have dismissed the case because it had worn on me emotionally. I had no idea until I requested the entire file, that Dr. Garland had falsified so many records in Robyn Edwards' medical file. Ben Mason had mentioned the inconsistencies but had never actually shown them to me.

Why would Nalder be attempting to file a case based on Garland not diagnosing MoyaMoya, when he was negligent of so many other things that were obvious: falsifying medical records, giving Zomig when he did not have a clear diagnosis and when he actually diagnosed a rare form of Migraine Headache? Robyn's primary care physician referred her over for numbness; there was no history of migraines in her file. So where did the history of Migraine headaches come from. Robyn saw Dr. Porter on August 25, 2007 and Dr. Garland on October 1, 2007, again where would the history of migraine headaches come from? Ben Mason had already pointed out the discrepancies, so why did Nalder not follow up?

3) On Page 2 of the letter from Nalder dated April 13, 2012, he states that Dr. XXX changed his position. He informed my ex-husband and I during the meeting on April 11, 2011 that Dr. XXX had recanted his statement and would not give anything in writing. Yet, he filed Dr. XXX's testimony in which Dr. XXX states Garland was gross negligent. If he indeed changed his position, why would Nalder proceed to file his testimony? Dr. XXX's testimony was filed in court on April 16, 2012. Consequently, I have attempted to contact Dr. XXX, but he will not return my calls. There is no way for me to know what transpired because no one knows what misinformation Nalder may have given him. Has anyone asked the expert witness if he actually retreated and why? The letter filed in court does not represent someone recanting or retreating.

Also, I in this age of technology, there are forensic document examiners. Robyn Edwards only saw Dr. Garland once. He added information to the notes after the initial notes were written, an examination will show this. Is that not a form of identifying if documents have been altered? Robyn saw Dr. Garland on October 1, 2007. She had the stroke on October 4. Garland had to have made the additions on October 5, 2007 or thereafter. Forensics can tell if the markings were made later.

4) The second reason Nalder gives is that they cannot prove when Robyn took the Zomig. Again, another falsehood on Nalder's part. The afternoon of October 4, 2007, Robyn took a Zomig, as we ate lunch at noon. I returned to work but was uncomfortable. I returned home about an hour later. It was about 2 in the afternoon. This is when Robyn began having the stroke symptoms and the onset of what we thought was a migraine headache but it was a stroke. I never changed my testimony because this is what happened. Nalder has intentionally attempted to undermine my testimony. This is the same statement I made to Ben Mason, during my deposition, and any other time I was questioned. There was only one time that I questioned myself because I considered giving Robyn another Zomig later on October 4, 2007 but I did not.

5) Why would an attorney not file the claim of one of the Plaintiffs? I recently realized that he did not file my claim in the case. I will forward a copy of all the expenses/claims he did file. Yes, he had all of my information. The only interest besides Robyn's and the experts was my ex-husband.

My ex-husband's attorney contacted Mr. Nalder after the meeting on April 11, 2012. After speaking with Nalder, he and my ex-husband wondered why Nalder did not like me. I have no clue. The only reason I can give is that about February, Nalder subpoenaed information regarding a discrimination complaint I filed in Idaho Falls in 2010. I wondered why he would allow this since he was representing me and the case was still in progress. I want you to know that they ruled against me. I do wonder if Nalder's request somehow affected their decision, giving them the impression that I am just out filing complaints against people. When in fact, I did not initiate the Malpractice Lawsuit, my ex-husband did. A discrimination complaint had no bearing on this Malpractice Lawsuit, why did Nalder allow such a thing? I was his client and he was supposed to be protecting my interest. He should have objected to this.

It was reiterated during the deposition that I had a claim. Terrence Jones requested my W-2's, pay history and employment information during the affected period. I submitted this information to Nalder. Is this another oversight on his part? Lance Nalder knew it would be difficult to find another attorney to represent a case in Idaho after one counsel withdrew. With Idaho Statute 6-1012, it is difficult to find one at all. So he knew when he withdrew, it would be almost impossible. He also knew that I was aware that the documents had been falsified because I identified this during the deposition. He also knew Robyn was turning 18 on June 24, 2012. So if he did not file my interest in the case, I would automatically be ruled out to represent the case, which is what happened. So my disabled daughter had to file Pro Se. We eventually dismissed without prejudice. I am not sure why Lance Nalder went to these extremes to sabotage my disabled daughter's case, but he did.

I also gave a copy of a manuscript I was working on "XXX" in which I encourage people, especially women, to stand up against injustice. Maybe this is what turned him against me. I honestly do not know. I do know that he was negligent and his actions unethical.

6) When Benjamin Mason left so did due diligence in fighting my disabled daughter's lawsuit. Lance Nalder proved through his own writings in the letter dated April 13, that he was giving the Plaintiffs misinformation. He was also aware that the documents in Robyn's medical records were altered and proceeded to use it to sabotage my testimony and mislead the expert witness.

7) I also noticed on several occasions that Mr. Nalder's office would send my personal information to my ex-husband but would not forward any of his information to me. For instance a copy of the Discrimination Complaint was forwarded to XXX, my ex-husband. When I called Nalder's office and asked, "Why?" I was told by XXX (a worker in his office) that my ex-husband had a right to it. So I then asked, "Well, where are my copies of the information he has submitted?" I was told she would check on it and get back to me. Of course no one ever got back to me on it.

I am a single, African American, Christian, Mother. I teach my children to follow the law and to be respectful of others. It is discouraging to know that there are people like Lance Nalder who use the law to manipulate and violate the rights of others. Lance Nalder and Breck Barton intentionally misled my ex-husband, the expert witness and attempted to intimidate me. Nalder used his knowledge of the discord between my ex-husband and me to his advantage. My ex-husband came to me and compelled me to take part in this lawsuit because of all the suffering our families had gone through and so that Robyn would have the resources to meet her needs in the future. This is not a vendetta. I forgave Dr. Garland a long time ago.

I ask you how Lance Nalder failed to file my claim? I brought Robyn home against the advice of the Medical Team at Primary Children's Hospital. They thought it would be too much for me to care for her at home. I resigned both my jobs and I lost the home I was planning to buy. My boys had to give up a lot of activities to assist in caring for Robyn. Robyn was total care when she came home. She could not walk, feed herself, toilet herself or dress herself. It took a year for her to walk again. I was her aid in Geometry in 11th grade because everyone else confused her. I did not work for almost three years and you mean with the knowledge of all of this, Lance Nalder somehow forgot to file a claim on my behalf? Lance Nalder used his knowledge of the legal system to abuse it.

I have a question for you all, why would he need to sabotage the case to withdraw? If the case was not viable, why threaten us that if we proceeded whether we won or loss he would come after us for his expenses? I understood that if we won he was entitled because of his expenses. If it was not viable, why the need to give misinformation to the plaintiffs, and the expert witness?

I never refused to pay Nalder. I requested an invoice the summer of 2012. I have not received another one. Also, I am not presently working. I moved to California so that Robyn could attend an Acquired Brain Injury Program. It was an act of faith but I do believe I will obtain employment and will address Nalder's invoice then. I do not plan to give in to these injustices. Lance Nalder's actions were negligent, unethical and blatant.

Enclosures:

a) *Copy of emails from Ben Mason to my ex-husband*
b) *Copy of Teton Radiology referral*

c) Coy of referral from Idaho Pediatrics to Dr. Garland
d) Copy of Actual Medical Expenses and Related Costs (from Nalder's files)
e) Copy of order denying request for summary judgment
f) Copy of letter stating Ben Mason left Nalder firm
g) Copy of letter regarding April 11th meeting to discuss Nalder's withdrawal from the case

Sincerely,
Veverly M Edwards
XXXX

After requesting a hearing before the Idaho Bar Professional Conduct Committee, the hearing was scheduled for April 13, 2013. During the recorded hearing, Mr. Nalder lied regarding knowledge of my claim in the malpractice lawsuit. His defense was that he never knew I had a claim because when he took the case over from Ben Mason, the only claims were that of my ex-husband and Robyn.

I also mentioned the falsified medical record in my complaint. Since it was not in the documents that were forwarded before the hearing, the committee asked me to forward these documents to them and that it was my last opportunity to send any documentation. When I forwarded the medical records, I also forwarded a copy of the deposition in which Mr. Nalder acknowledged my claim in the case.

In addition, I sent the requested medical document which was written in Dr. Garland's handwriting. Mr. Nalder referenced it in his letter to withdraw as the evidence that shows that I admitted to Robyn having migraine headaches. According to Mr. Nalder, of course this compromised my testimony. Now, just looking at the document, anyone can distinguish the fact that the writing on the document in question is not mine. To support this fact, I had the document examined by a forensic document expert.

In March of 2013, I made the sacrifice to pay to have a forensic document examiner analyze the medical record to determine whose handwriting was on the document in question. I sent in the document, along with other documents I filled out in Dr. Garland's office on October 1, 2007, and the documents in the file with his handwriting. Sure enough, the document Mr. Nalder claimed compromised my testimony is not in my handwriting. Imagine that! The forensic document examiner's opinion is on the next page.

April 18, 2013

Case # 13-105

Prepared for:

Veverly Edwards

Opinion Letter

Jill Wilson
Court-Qualified, Certified Forensic Document Examiner
3943 Irvine Boulevard #42
Irvine, CA 92602-2400
714-642-3016

Case # 13-105
This letter contains a statement of the request of the client, descriptions of the questioned and exemplar documents, a synopsis of the examination conducted, and this document examiner's opinion.

1.0 Request

I was asked to compare known writing of Veverly Edwards and known writing of Erich W. Garland MD (see "Description of the Exemplar Documents" on page 2) to writing on the questioned document (see "Description of the Questioned Document") to determine the following:

- Does the writing on the questioned document belong to Veverly Edwards?
- Could Erich W. Garland MD have authored the writing on the questioned document?

I received electronic documents (PDF and JPG files) by e-mail from Veverly Edwards on April 17, 2013.

2.0 Description of the Questioned Document

I examined the following questioned document (labeled copy enclosed):

Q1. Review of Systems, dated 10/1/07, "Garland 00028" appears in lower right corner

The only writing on the questioned document is "*Robyn Edwards*" on the NAME line, "*10/1/07*" on the DATE line, and "*NA*" on each of the "number of pregnancies," "last Pap smear," and "last mammogram" lines. Additionally, the following items are circled in the NEUROLOGIC section at the bottom of the form: Dizziness, numbness, weakness, balance, changes in speech, headaches.

3.0 Description of the Exemplar Documents

I examined the following exemplar documents (scanned, JPG) bearing known writing of Veverly Edwards (labeled copies enclosed):

KV1. Idaho Falls Neurology Patient Information form for Robyn Edwards, dated 10-01-07

KV2. Idaho Falls Neurology Health History form for Robyn Edwards, dated 10/01/07

KV3. Worker's Compensation form, dated 10/01/07

I examined the following exemplar documents (PDF) bearing known writing of Erich W. Edwards MD (labeled copies enclosed):

KG1. History of Present Illness form for Robyn Edwards, dated 10-1-07, marked Garland 00055

KG2. Medication Record for Robyn Edwards, dated 10/1/07, marked Garland 00029

KG3. Neurological Examination form for Robyn Edwards, dated 10-1-07, marked Garland 00057

KG4. Impressions/Decisions/Plans form for Robyn Edwards, dated 10-1-07, marked Garland 00058

KG5. Photocopy of 4 prescription slips for Robyn Edwards, dated 10/1/07, marked Garland 00027

KG6. Physician Referral form for Robyn Edwards, Date of Service 10/9/07, marked Garland 00062

4.0 Examination

The basis for handwriting identification is that writing habits are not instinctive or hereditary but are complex processes that are developed gradually through habit, and that handwriting is unique to each individual. Further, the basic axiom is that no one person writes exactly the same way twice and no two people write exactly the same. Thus, writing habits or individual characteristics distinguish one person's handwriting from another's.

A process of analysis, comparison, and evaluation is conducted between the known standards (exemplar documents) and the questioned documents. This process adheres to ASTM[1] E-2290, "Standard Guide for Examination of Handwritten Items." The conclusions of the expert opinions are derived from ASTM E-1658, "Standard Terminology for Expressing Conclusions for Forensic Document Examiners."

I apply accepted forensic document examination tools, principles, and techniques to analyze the documents submitted to me for inspection and to compare details of the writing on all questioned documents to each other as well as against the writing on the exemplar documents.

1. American Society for Testing and Materials

5.0 Opinion

Based on a thorough analysis of the documents submitted to me, my professional expert opinion is as follows:

- Owing to significant differences, as well as a lack of significant similarities, observed between the known writing of Veverly Edwards and the questioned writing on Q1 (all from 10/1/07), Veverly Edwards is eliminated as the author of the writing on Q1.
- Owing to significant similarities observed between the known writing of Erich W. Garland MD and the questioned writing on Q1 (all but one from 10/1/07), Erich W. Garland MD is identified as the author of the writing on Q1. Further, there is evidence to suggest that Erich W. Garland MD circled the items in the NEUROLOGIC section at the bottom of the form.

6.0 Declarations and Signature

I am willing to testify to this fact in a court of law and to present evidence to support my opinion.

I declare under penalty of perjury under the laws of the state of California that the foregoing is true and correct.

Respectfully submitted,

Jill Wilson

Jill Wilson
Certified Forensic Document Examiner

April 18, 2013

Although I did not have the forensic document examiner's opinion as of the date of the hearing, it is evident by viewing the document that it is not in my handwriting. My question has always been, 'what compensation are these individuals receiving for them to compromise themselves?" They are determined to undermine me. What is worse is that the organizations which supposedly are there for recourse for complaints against those abusing their licenses, ignore the evidence presented to them, and rule in favor of the licensee regardless of the offense.

After sending in the information to the Idaho Bar Professional Conduct Committee, I received a letter a few weeks later. In their opinion Mr. Nalder "properly preformed his duties." Their final opinion is on the next page.

PROFESSIONAL CONDUCT BOARD
P.O. Box 895
Boise, Idaho 83701

**BEFORE THE PROFESSIONAL CONDUCT BOARD
OF THE IDAHO STATE BAR**

IN THE MATTER OF G. LANCE NALDER, Attorney at Law.	ISB CASE NO. 12-187a APPEAL/REVIEW COMMITTEE DECISION

This matter came before the duly appointed Appeal/Review Committee on Complainant's request for review of the disposition of the Office of Bar Counsel, dated March December 14, 2012, pursuant to Idaho Bar Commission Rule 509(d). The Appeal/Review Committee has reviewed the record before it. The Complainant requested a hearing, which has held on March 12, 2013. The Appeal/Review Committee allowed the Complainant to submit additional evidence for consideration after the hearing, which was received on March 19, 2013.

This request for review concerns whether the attorney, G. Lance Nalder, violated the Idaho Rules of Professional Conduct in his representation of Veverly Edwards, Robert Edwards and Robyn Edwards (the former's disabled daughter). Specifically, Complainant contends that Mr. Nalder violated the Idaho Rules of Professional Conduct by withdrawing from his representation of the family group with respect to claims he had been advancing on their behalf for medical negligence.

Deputy Bar Counsel determined that the Complainant's allegations implicated Rules 1.2 and 1.16(d) of the Idaho Rules of Professional Conduct. After performing an investigation, Deputy Bar Counsel concluded that the Complainant had failed to carry her burden of proof that Mr. Nalder had violated the Idaho Rules of Professional Conduct.

The Appeal/Review Committee has considered the evidence in the record, in light of the fact that the burden of proof is upon the Complainant to establish a violation of the Idaho Rules of Professional Conduct by clear and convincing evidence. *See* Rule 522(f), Idaho Rules of Professional Conduct. In addition, the Appeal/Review Committee has considered the comments and testimony of the Complainant and Mr. Nalder at the hearing. The Appeal/Review Committee has also reviewed and considered the evidence submitted by Complainant after the hearing. The Appeal/Review Committee finds that there is no clear and convincing evidence that Mr. Nalder violated the Rules in his representation of Complainant and her family members or in his dealings with the Complainant and her family members. It is the opinion of the Appeal/Review Committee that Mr. Nalder properly performed all obligations he owed to Complainant and her family members, under the Idaho Rules of Professional Conduct, incident to his withdrawal as their attorney.

Now, therefore, IT IS THE UNANIMOUS DECISION OF THE APPEAL COMMITTEE that the disposition of the Office of the Bar Counsel be **APPROVED**.

DATED this 27th day of March, 2013.

PROFESSIONAL CONDUCT BOARD

David P. Claiborne
Chairman of Appeal/Review Committee

APPEAL/REVIEW COMMITTEE DECISION - Page 2

About a month or so after the hearing, I finally had the opportunity to speak with the expert witness and he denied making any changes to his testimony. As a matter of fact, he stated that if he had changed anything it would have been in writing. Mr. Nalder shared with him that I had compromised my testimony by acknowledging that Robyn had headaches and that it was, now, impossible to determine how many Zomig tablets Robyn had taken. Dr. XXX never changed his position. But because Mr. Nalder asked, he did tell Mr. Nalder that given this new information it may make the case more difficult. Dr. XXX also stated that he would still be available to give his testimony if I continued with the case. Consequently, the expert witness concluded that Dr. Garland was gross negligent in his care of Robyn. The expert's eight-page testimony is in the appendix section.

After reading the initial opinion of the Idaho Bar Association and the final opinion of the Professional Conduct Committee, I believe they were letting me know that regardless of the evidence, they were going to rule in his favor. Mr. Nalder lied about the expert's opinion, lied regarding my claim, lied about me compromising my testimony, and the Idaho Bar Association's Professional Conduct Committee found that he properly performed his duties.

I honestly believe that Mr. Nalder, Dr. Garland and all the organizations and officials who have taken part in this cover up thought I would eventually give in to their tactics. I refuse to give in because I have God and the truth on my side. Earlier this year (2013), when I contacted the expert witness on the case, he verbally informed me that he did not change his testimony. Of course, according to Mr. Nalder's letter he repositioned himself after Dr. Garland's attorney supposedly found an Idaho doctor who challenged Dr. XXX's testimony. When I asked for the name of this Idaho expert who supposedly challenged our expert, Attorney Barton refused to give his name during the meeting in April of 2012.

Mr. Nalder succeeded in blocking me from speaking to our expert in 2012. As you have already read in the letter, Mr. Nalder wrote stating that Dr. XXX would not speak to me unless Mr. Nalder was allowed to withdraw from the case. The letter also suggested that I would have to pay Dr. XXX, if I wanted any additional information regarding his testimony. Well, that was a lie too. It became apparent that Mr. Nalder included the money issue to further discourage me from contacting the expert. When I finally spoke with Dr. XXX, the earlier part of 2013, he stated that he never changed his testimony.

While the judge presiding over Robyn's malpractice case, the Idaho Bar Association, the Idaho Falls Police, and the FBI refused to investigate my complaint regarding Mr. Nalder defrauding a case he was representing, I did not allow that to hinder me from continuing to gather information. On October 30, 2013, I wrote the expert. I forwarded a copy of the letter Mr. Nalder wrote to me on April 13, 2012, stating that he had changed his position. I specifically asked Dr. XXX to provide in writing what he stated to me earlier in the year. That he had not changed his statement and had he changed it he would have done so in writing. The expert's response is on the following page.

DIPLOMATE AMERICAN BOARD OF
NEUROLOGY

MEDICAL NEUROLOGY
ELECTROENCEPHALOGRAPHY
ELECTROMYOGRAPHY

November 11, 2013

TO WHOM IT MAY CONCERN **RE:** Edward, Robyn v Garland

On 1/11/10 and again on 3/22/12 I dictated reports to Benjamin Mason, Esq. Law offices of Nalder Law Office 591 Park Avenue , Suite 201 Idaho Falls, ID 83402, concerning my review of records and opinion with regards to Robyn Edwards. Additionally I signed an affidavit and a supplemental affidavit concerning this case on 11/22/10 and 2/8/11 respectively. The purpose of this letter is to confirm that my opinions expressed in those documents has not changed. Specifically I have not "recanted", "retreated" or "repositioned" my opinion. If I had done so I would have done so in writing. I am still willing to be an expert witness in this matter through the attorney for Robyn Edwards.

Sincerely,

If the Bar Association used Mr. Nalder's statement regarding the expert witness as fact, and I questioned it, and provided written documents showing the inconsistency, why did they not see the contradictions in his actions? During the April 11, 2012 meeting, Mr. Nalder told us nothing existed in writing and the expert had recanted or repositioned his statement. Yet, he filed the expert's testimony on April 16, 2012. By the way, this was also the deadline he gave us to withdraw without being charged his fees too. Had I withdrawn, the expert's testimony probably would have never been filed and the entire case would have been dismissed with prejudice. Does that not sound suspicious? Not to the Idaho Bar Association.

During the hearing on May 30, 2012 for Mr. Nalder's motion to withdraw from the case, I pleaded with Judge Tingey to discontinue the civil case and turn the case over for criminal investigation because Mr. Nalder, Mr. Barton and Dr. Garland had falsified medical documents in the case. Judge Tingey denied my request. If these individuals and boards wanted the truth, they could have simply called the expert, and he would have provided it at that time. Mr. Nalder and Mr. Barton, who purportedly represented our interests, provided distorted information about me to others to keep the case from going forward. They succeeded because no one would listen nor examine the truth that was in writing

In the Idaho Bar Association's interpretation of my initial complaint, they said that I implied that Mr. Nalder violated Idaho Professional Rules of Conduct (I.P.R.C.) 1.2 and 1.16. I.P.R.C. 1.2 relates to the decisions regarding the objectives of the case. 1.16 is in regard to termination of representation. What the Idaho Bar failed to acknowledge is the bigger issue of fraud and deception on Mr. Nalder's part which relates to I.P.R.C. 8.4 Misconduct.

According to rule 8.4 Misconduct, it is misconduct for a lawyer to engage in fraud or deceit, engage in an act that is prejudicial to the administration of justice, and to improperly influence a government agency or official to achieve results that violate the Rules of Professional Conduct or other law.

Mr. Nalder committed fraud. He lied on the expert witness. Now, I would think, since the Idaho Bar Association took Mr. Nalder's written statement as truth in their first response to my complaint, that they would have talked to the expert witness and verified Mr. Nalder's statement. According to the first letter from the Idaho Bar, in their opinion, my complaint was unfounded. They acknowledged my complaint regarding Mr. Nalder's lie regarding the expert witness, but found nothing wrong with his behavior.

I also sent the Idaho Bar the letter Nalder wrote on April 13, 2012, stating that the expert witness had retreated from his previous opinion, and a copy of the expert witness testimony which was filed with the court on April 16, 2012. The Idaho Bar saw no inconsistency with this action. If an expert recants or changes his position on his testimony, is the testimony still filed with the court without any mention of changes? Mr. Nalder filed the testimony that the expert witness supposedly recanted and the Bar saw nothing suspicious with this action.

In a letter dated May 9, 2012, Mr. Nalder made it clear that the expert witness was not going to communicate with me. I sent that letter to the Bar too. Now, had the Idaho Bar Association actually investigated my complaint, they would have found out that Dr. XXX never recanted, repositioned, nor retreated in any way from the testimony he gave Mr. Nalder.

On March 12, 2013, during a recorded hearing before the Professional Conduct Committee, Mr. Nalder lied. Yet, they saw nothing wrong with his actions. One of my concerns in my second letter to the Idaho Bar Association was Mr. Nalder's failure to file my claim in the case. During the recorded hearing, Mr. Nalder stated that he was not aware that I had a claim in the case. I sent the Idaho Bar Association's Professional Conduct Committee a copy of a page from the deposition where Mr. Nalder acknowledges my claim. I also sent a letter that Mr. Nalder sent to me requesting financial and tax information necessary to file my claim. Again, the committee saw nothing wrong with Mr. Nalder's action.

My concern with the Idaho Bar Association is that even with the inconsistencies in Mr. Nalder's statements and filings with the court, they found that he "properly performed" his duties to my family and me. Was Mr. Nalder's actions really representative of the Idaho Bar Association?

Chapter 5

Our Challenges in California

30 Moreover whom he did predestinate, them he also called: and whom he called, them he also justified: and whom he justified, them he also glorified.
31 What shall we then say to these things? If God be for us, who can be against us?

Romans 8:30-31, (KJV)

October 23, 2012, as I maneuvered out of bed, I prayed that the pain was gone for good. Robyn was calling, "Mama, can you help me put my blouse on now?" I was told yesterday by a physician at Hoag Hospital's emergency room that I should stay off my feet for a couple of days. It appears that I have irritated the sciatic nerve in my lower back. I wanted to tell the doctor that staying off my feet for a couple of days was not an option, but instead I asked to speak with a social worker. I had tried every agency referred to me. Now, I thought, maybe, the hospital could help.

"Hi, is your name Veverly?" the thin blonde asked, as she approached me.

"Yes, it is," I replied.

"That's such a pretty name. Never heard of Veverly. Did you request to speak
with a social worker," she asked?

"I did." She then introduced herself to me and I extended my hand.

"How can I help you?"

"Well, not sure if you can. My family and I moved here in August. I came here so that my disabled daughter could attend an Acquired Brain Injury Program. She had a stroke at 13-years-old. I resigned my job in Idaho Falls, Idaho and moved to Costa Mesa. It has been difficult. For a while we lived with a relative in San Gabriel. I took the last of my savings and used it to stay at the Howard Johnson Inn, in Orange, California, while I searched for a job. Now that has run out and I still haven't found a job or a place for us to live."

"Your daughter had a stroke at 13-years-old?"

"Yeah, due to a condition called MoyaMoya." *I decided not to add that a doctor gave a drug that caused mini strokes to become a massive stroke and that she was actually pronounced brain dead on October 9, 2007...*

"Yeah, and she is the reason I moved here, to attend a Brain Injury Program.

"Oh, so your stay will run out soon?"

"No, actually my stay ran out several weeks ago. I was wondering, if you could refer my family and me somewhere for assistance?"

"Oh, I'm sorry. I don't have a lot of shelters that I can refer you to. The only ones I have are the overnight kind that you have to stand in line for each day."

Lying on my back, the pain medicine started to kick in, I knew that standing in line would not be on my list today. She handed me the list of shelters.

"Sorry, I know this probably won't be of much help."

"Thanks. I appreciate whatever you can do." I took the list.

"I hope you find something," she said, as she exited the room.

Well, at least I had a couple of uninterrupted hours lying down in bed. I wanted to ask for a couple more hours, but I did not. Instead, I leaned back, inhaled the smell of the disinfectants in the air, which reminded me of my second home. One of the memories that stick out in my mind about Primary Children's Hospital, is how clean it was. Robyn and I lived there for five months, and it actually became a place of comfort.

I was given a pain pill to help with the pain and was thankful for that. I looked at my older son, slumped over on the counter with a pillow under his head. I felt guilty. I resigned a decent job and moved him and his siblings to California. I was naïve to think that I could possibly find a job in a few weeks or even a couple of months. My children do not seem to be bothered by the fact that we have no place to call home. However, I am ready to go home to Tennessee, where my mother and support systems are.

"Mama," Robyn called again.

"I'm on my way." *Well at least my back feels better this morning*. I walked slowly into the adjoining bathroom. I helped Robyn with her blouse. I looked at her feet. "We'll have to put your shoe and brace on in the bedroom because I need to be sitting." After assisting her, she went downstairs to get breakfast. I turned and looked at the unmade bed. As I walked over to make it, I could feel the pain starting to move across my hips. I wanted to crawl back under the warm comfort of the blanket, but time would not permit. I slowly pulled the sheets and comforter across the king-sized bed, being careful not to make any sudden moves. With each step I took, I could feel the nerve endings awakening. Once I completed the task, I sat for a moment contemplating my next move. I really needed to sit in a hot tub of water which usually helped with my pain management.

As I dressed, I realized how late it was. If we were going to get from San Gabriel to Costa Mesa in time for my youngest son's first class, we needed to leave now. So much for staying off my feet for a couple of days, oh, and not driving is just not an option for a single mom. Although I understand why I should not drive, every bump in the road is just a reminder of how painful it is to irritate the sciatic nerve.

After I dropped my youngest son off and wrote a letter explaining that his mom's injured back was the reason for him being absent, I took Robyn to school. Consequently, his school did not accept the letter and questioned the validity of it because I was supposed to write a letter explaining why he was late, not absent.

No matter how bad I feel and how many times I second guess the move, when I see how well they have adjusted, I know that it is worth the struggle. My son is now on the cross-country team at his school. Robyn is excited every morning she arrives at school. The first week she attended school, she said, "Mom, it felt so good walking across campus. I felt independent. I never thought this would happen for me. I felt free."

The Acquired Brain Injury Program has given Robyn something I could not give her. I remember, in the spring, she passed the initial assessment for entrance into the program. She came home and posted on her Facebook page, "I feel so good that there is a place for people like me." Everyone had posted where they were going for college and now she could post too. That made my heart smile. I am in a precarious position, homeless, no job, but happy kids.

As we loaded into the car, I saw the letter I refused to give attention to yesterday: addressed to Veverly and Robyn Edwards from Bonneville County Civil Court, Idaho Falls, Idaho. I grabbed it and held on to it as I drove. I will read it after I drop them off at school. I feel more resolute today. Yesterday, my resolve was low, and I was in a lot of pain. As I drove, I wondered if the judge considered our last request.

This entire situation is surreal, from Robyn's stroke to me representing a medical malpractice lawsuit. Why would Robyn's attorney undermine her Malpractice lawsuit? What kind of doctor changes the medical records of a child he nearly killed? What kind of court system will see the injustice and not respond? When I recall the conversations and events of the April 11, 2012 meeting, I am simply stumped. I know they lied and that is why I cannot walk away.

"...Mr. and Ms. Edwards the expert witness recanted his earlier statements once he knew we had a neurologist in Boise that challenged his testimony...," stated Mr. Nalder.

As my ex-husband asked questions over the phone, I watched Mr. Nalder and Mr. Barton.

I interrupted, "I thought you couldn't find a neurologist to speak to the standard of care. When Ben Mason was representing us, he said that everyone had either taken a vow of silence or refused to return his calls. How did you get one to come forward?"

"I have contacts in Boise and a neurologist that I know spoke to me off record...," said Barton.

"Can you show me something in writing from our expert witness," I asked?

"No, I cannot. He has refused to give anything in writing," Nalder replied.

"Well, wasn't he paid to give something in writing?" I continued.

"Ms. Edwards that is not the only issue. You filled out paperwork that compromised your testimony..."

"No, I didn't. What paperwork?" Nalder slid a paper before me which I had previously seen at the deposition. "Hold on. That is not my handwriting." When I reached for it, he snatched it back. "Mr. Nalder that is the same document that Dr. Garland's attorney presented to me during my deposition and I told him it was not my handwriting. You were there."

"There is also the fact that we cannot establish when Robyn took the medication the day of her stroke..."

I was speechless, in total amazement. I know that he knew I was aware of his deception.

Mr. Barton interrupted. "Ms. Edwards I understand how you feel. I had a son who had a birth injury, and we too thought the doctor was at fault, but after a lot of agony my wife and I realized that sometimes bad things happen, and we need someone to blame; so we take it out on the doctor... We finally let go and moved on...," he stated.

"Mr. Barton, I got passed my anger a long time ago or I wouldn't have made it this far. I am grateful to God that He spared Robyn's life. She is alive only by His grace. I didn't even initiate the lawsuit, my ex-husband did. I am not even concerned with Dr. Garland at this point. I am more concerned with what is going on in this room." I leaned back in my chair, crossed my arms and just stared. They took on a different appearance to me. They now appeared to me as beaded-eyed devils in business suits, attempting to deceive and intimidate me to dismiss the case with prejudice.

Mr. Nalder was pacing the floor, "You're not gonna win! You're not gonna win!" he exploded. I did not respond; I just watched him. My ex-husband continued to try and make sense out of what they were saying. After watching them both, I knew something else had transpired that we were not privy to.

Mr. Nalder went on to explain that if we dismissed now, he would forgive his fees, and was sure he could get the defendant's side to forgive their fees too. My ex-husband was listening on speaker phone. Mr. Nalder wanted us to decide in his office. "You and I need to discuss this further in private before making a decision," I stated to my ex-husband.

"Also, you two don't have to agree. One could dismiss and the other could continue. I would still forgive the fees of the one that dismisses," Nalder stated. However, if you don't dismiss, I will expect my fees whether you win or lose if you continue with the case."

"Wait, so you are saying that if we find counsel and continue with the case, after you have withdrawn, you will expect to be paid, whether we win or lose," I asked.

"Yes," replied Mr. Nalder.

"When do you need to have our answer," I asked. Mr. Nalder wanted us to make a decision during the meeting.

"By noon on Monday, April 16th," replied Mr. Barton.

As I left the building, I was in shock, not because they withdrew, but because they had used false information, and had attempted to defraud us. This only happens in movies, right? I sent a text to my ex-husband.

"You know they are lying, right?"

"I don't understand, why are they concentrating on the registration form at the doctor's office? She was referred to him for numbness in her limbs not migraine headaches," my ex-husband, replied.

"Do you think someone may have paid them off? Nalder knows that I didn't fill out that form. My bad handwriting is very distinguishable and Nalder has a copy of all the documents."

"I need to discuss this with my lawyer. I will be in contact later," stated my ex-husband.

"Well, I'm not giving in to them. If he lied about my handwriting, chances are he is lying on the expert witness too."

That evening, I went home and tried to piece the puzzle together. The weekend before the April meeting, the kids and I were in California on their spring break. While there I received a call from Attorney Lane Blake, an attorney working with Mr. Nalder on Robyn's case. I was told that a Life Planner they hired had tried to contact me. They needed to submit the life plan assessment on Robyn in court on Monday, April 2, 2012. I left California early to make it home in time for the Life Planner to come by the house to do the assessment on Sunday, April 1, 2012.

Several weeks before we left for California, Attorney Blake called me into the office because they were trying to contact a doctor from Primary Children's Hospital to obtain information regarding Robyn's condition. He said nothing whatsoever about any problems. I had also made an appointment to speak with Mr. Nalder regarding filing guardianship over Robyn because she was about to turn 18-years-old and was not ready to take on adult responsibilities. I made the appointment for April 3, 2012. I was told that Mr. Nalder would be out of town for two weeks. That was fine because it would be after we returned.

I do recall a letter coming in the mail from Mr. Nalder, stating that we needed to meet regarding the case. When Robyn and I met with Mr. Nalder on April 3, 2012, he informed me that he could not represent me in filing guardianship over Robyn. It would be a conflict of interest since he was representing both her father and me in the malpractice lawsuit. So, he referred me to another attorney. He also stated that he had some concerns with the case and that he wanted to schedule a meeting with my ex-husband and me. He went on to say that I had stated that Robyn had headaches on some medical forms.

"No I did not, because she did not have headaches. She had numbing sensations," I stated.

He then leaned in towards the table, "What is Robyn's life expectancy," he asked? I felt like I was about to explode, but Robyn was now watching me and waiting for my response.

"What do you mean? What is her life expectancy? She has no limits on her life."

"Well, I need to meet with you and Mr. Edwards. I have scheduled the meeting for April 11, 2012.

"Nice meeting you Mr. Nalder," Robyn said, as we walked out. I was still livid. When we walked outside, Robyn stopped and looked at me.

"Mom, am I gonna die?"

"Robyn, we are all going to die."

"You know what I mean."

"Yes, I do, and if someone had placed a limit on your life, do you think I wouldn't have told you? The only limit placed on your life was when the doctors pronounced you brain dead and did not think you would make it through the week of October 9, 2007."

"God and I proved them wrong, huh?"

"Yes, and the only one that knows any of our limits is God." I could not believe Mr. Nalder would do such a thing. When I arrived home, I checked my missed calls and saw that Robyn's primary care physician had called. That was not normal. So, I called the office back. The receptionist checked her files. She said that Lance Nalder had called Robyn's doctor wanting to know Robyn's life expectancy.

"What did Dr. Moore say," I asked?

"The note states that he informed Mr. Nalder, that there is no life expectancy on Robyn," she replied.

The more I thought about the past weeks the more confused I was. My mind raced. How is Mr. Nalder benefiting? I never thought he would attempt to defraud us as he has. What is his motivation? Politics? Money? I wondered with the present political climate and the fact that Dr. Garland was well known among the community of neurologists and because of the positions he held, if someone had paid Mr. Nalder off to undermine the case. It just did not add up. I never met Mr. Barton until April 11, 2012. What was his role in the deception and how did he profit?

Well, I already knew that I was not going to dismiss the case. I also knew that Mr. Nalder and Mr. Barton were lying. A couple of days after the meeting, I requested Robyn's medical files from Dr. Garland's office. At first, they refused to give them to me, until I informed them that under HIPPA I had a right to copies of Robyn's files. They stated that they had already given copies to my attorney, but I stated I did not have a copy. They finally agreed but said it would take two to three days because they were in storage.

On Monday, April 16, I called Nalder's office and requested copies of the medical records they received from Dr. Garland. Of course, they sent me a partial file. Dr. Garland's office called me on April 17, 2012, and told me I could pick up the information. Needless to say it was not what I requested but I eventually received the files.

Dr. Garland falsified the diagnosis and the symptoms. He added migraine headache as the diagnosis and said that Robyn sometimes had headaches that lasted all day. The importance of the headaches and the diagnosis is that he gave Robyn a medication, Zomig, which is given for migraine headaches. He actually, diagnosed her with a rare form of migraine and gave Zomig to treat it. Robyn never had a headache with the numbing sensation prior to taking the medication. The only symptoms she experienced were numbness in her limbs. She was actually having mini strokes because the condition she had, MoyaMoya, causes the carotid arteries to slowly occlude. The Zomig made them constrict and close, causing a massive stroke.

I kept asking myself whether he did it intentionally. Why and when did he change her medical records? Robyn was a happy 13-year-old African American teenager. Did he not think she deserved the same diligence in care and diagnostic testing to insure her medical safety as a white teen? Everything I have read about the drug, since her stroke, says not to give it unless you are sure of your diagnosis. There was even an article that came out in the earlier part of 2007 stating that it was not recommended for children. Was he just using it for marketing to help pharmaceuticals?

During my search through her files, I found a letter dated October 1, 2007, to Dr. Porter the referring physician, and it too included migraine headaches in several paragraphs. He also stated in the letter that he and I had agreed on ordering an MRI. The truth, I ordered the MRI the day after the appointment and the MRI was confirmed the third of October, and Dr. Garland's signature is on the document dated the third. So, there is no way he could have included it in the letter written on the first of October.

Now, Attorney Nalder and Barton, tried to convince me that Dr. Garland was innocent and this bad thing just happened because of Robyn's pre-existing condition. I guess the "what is her life expectancy" question was to try and make a case that she was going to die anyway and to somehow explain away what Dr. Garland did to her.

Before Mr. Nalder took over the case, Ben Mason, another attorney with Mr. Nalder's Law Firm, was representing the case. He left in the earlier part of 2011. He never told us he was leaving.

We received a letter from Nalder's office that he was gone. At the time, I was too bogged down with my kids and I just let it stay with Nalder. But before Mr. Mason left, he informed me that during the deposition with Dr. Garland, it was obvious that he did not have enough information in his files to even speak to the care he gave Robyn. He certainly did not have the same perception as Mr. Nalder and Mr. Barton. The following is a letter that Robyn's father forwarded to me from Mr. Mason:

> *I wanted to write quickly and let you know how the deposition of Dr. Garland went. He was evasive in the areas where I thought he would be, and flat refused to answer some pertinent questions until he was pressed. The upshot is that (a) he is claiming that the local standard for Idaho Falls board-certified neurologists is not the same as the national standard, but is in fact whatever he personally chooses it to be. He said he never consults with other local neurologists and doesn't know what they do or don't do. He said that there was nothing unusual about Robyn's migraines, even though he wrote "unusual migraines" on her report, and "atypical migraine" on the prescription sheet for the MRI. He said that the MRI, even if he'd done it immediately, wouldn't have revealed the problem, even though he admits that when the ER doctor did the MRI it revealed an abnormality which led to them doing a CT and then a CT Angiogram, which is what revealed the MoyaMoya, which Dr. Garland diagnoses from the imaging. Anyway, the next step is to get the deposition transcript to our expert, Dr. XXX, and see if he thinks the statements made by Dr. Garland are enough for Dr. XXX to say that he is familiar with the local standard of care. If not, we'll continue trying to find another local guy.*
> *Ben*

It appears after Mr. Mason left, so did the due diligence needed in fighting Robyn's case.

The expert witness, which Mr. Mason retained, was a licensed medical examiner from California. He wrote in his conclusion that Dr. Garland was not only negligent but was gross negligent. He was not informed of the fact that the medical files he received had been falsified. So I guess, with all of Dr. Garland's energy to falsify the records, an expert in his field still found his actions to be negligent.

After the meeting with Mr. Nalder and Barton on April 11, 2012, I sprung into my own investigation. I went home and opened letters from Nalder that I had not opened. I generally called and received an overview from them as to what was transpiring. I had so much going on with the children, just trying to keep them focused, that I placed all my trust in Mr. Nalder's Law Firm to do what was right regarding the medical malpractice lawsuit.

Once I had the files of Dr. Garland, I requested the medical records from Robyn's primary care physician. A co-worker and I went to lunch and searched through the files to see if we could find any inconsistencies. Of course there were many with Dr. Garland's files. For example, there was the note that he wrote on October 1, 2007, in which he added headache symptoms; he even embellished it to the point of stating Robyn had headaches that sometimes lasted all day. He also added a phone number and name to this record. I called the number. It was to Primary Children's Hospital Neuro Intensive Care Unit and the name was that of a doctor who was on Robyn's medical team. Robyn was airlifted to Primary Children's Hospital on October 5, 2007. She only saw Dr. Garland once in his office and then in the emergency room at Eastern Idaho Regional Medical Center.

Several days after ordering Robyn's medical files, one of my co-workers gave me a copy of a magazine article that appeared in the Post Register Newspaper in Idaho Falls, Idaho. The front page had a picture of Dr. Garland and an article regarding the Joint Commission giving an award regarding Garland's and Eastern Idaho Regional Medical Center's stroke awareness and care. After reading the article, I began pacing the floor.

"Veverly, calm down" my co-worker stated as he turned around towards me.

"I can't believe this. He caused my child to stroke and nearly die. She laid in ERMIC for almost 12 hours or more before they even diagnosed it, and they are being given an award for early intervention practices!" I continued to pace the floor.

"Calm down. Have you found another attorney to take the case?"

I stopped, with my hands on my hips, "No, because everyone wants to know if I have a doctor that will establish the standard of care."

"Have you tried the ones I suggested?"

"I did, but they don't have anyone in this area. I have tried top law firms even in New York, but the best ones don't have anyone in this area to represent their firm." I took the magazine insert and began reading more on the article. "Do you think this could be tied to why Nalder and Barton attempted to defraud us and withdrew from the case?"

"It could be, you never know."

"I imagine the Joint Commission wasn't aware that he had a lawsuit pending for causing a 13-year-old to have a stroke by prescribing the wrong medication. I bet you, this has something to do with Nalder withdrawing and trying to intimidate us into dismissing. I imagine money is coming in to the hospital for some kind of stroke awareness initiative, and Dr. Garland is connected to it."

"Could be, but we need to get to work on this project." I sat at my desk and worked through the distraction the article had caused. Every now and then, I would turn to my co-worker, "Who do they think they are?"

"Girl stay focused. Get back to work," he replied.

My ex-husband decided to dismiss his interest in the case. He had an attorney from Memphis to call Mr. Nalder. Mr. Nalder expressed the same lie to his attorney that he gave us. He said Mr. Nalder also went on and on about the EEO complaint I filed against a Federal Contractor in Idaho. His attorney questioned Mr. Nalder's attitude towards me. Since my ex-husband had nothing in writing and no one knew whether the expert witness had actually recanted, his attorney advised him to dismiss.

Since I did not dismiss Robyn's and my interest in the case, on April 16, 2012, Mr. Nalder had to file paperwork with the court regarding the experts that would testify in the case. A week or so later, I received copies of the documents. Mr. Nalder filed the testimony of the expert witness that he told us had recanted his statement.

The expert witness wrote an eight-page testimony. After examining records and depositions, he came to the conclusion that Dr. Garland was gross negligent in his care of Robyn. The letter was signed March 28, 2012, several weeks before Mr. Nalder met with my ex-husband and me. Consequently, a week before I received these documents, I received a letter in writing regarding the meeting on April 11, 2007, and my options. Of course, the written document was vague and not reflective of what he told us in the meeting. Instead of stating that the expert recanted in the letter, Mr. Nalder stated that he changed his position. Instead of referencing the false medical record he presented in the office as having my handwriting on it, he simply states that I compromised my testimony by stating she had headaches. Lastly, he stated that I was unable to state when Robyn took the Zomig which was also a lie.

I had about forty-five days before we were to appear in court for his plea to withdraw as counsel. Well, this was taking place in the midst of Robyn's graduation activities. Several months earlier, I was asked to be the keynote speaker for the Baccalaureate Service. I was excited and honored that the class president and her mom thought enough of me to ask. Robyn was asked to do the closing prayer. We also had to find a prom dress and wrap up assignments. I had family coming in for her graduation.

Meanwhile, my oldest son was flying home from school, and I had to make his reservations. My fifteen-year-old son also had end-of-the-year activities. Now, finding another attorney was added to the list.

During my lunch break, I would go to the car and make calls to law firms. My company had disbanded the use of cell phones in the office. So, yet, another challenge, though a small one, but with everything else I was dealing with, I could not tell. Call after call and disappointment after disappointment, still no one to represent Robyn's interest in the case.

It was almost impossible for me to concentrate at work, but I had a friend that continued to needle me and would not let me fall into despair. Thank God for Christian friends/co-workers. In the evenings, I went home and forced myself to work on my speech which was now beginning to feel like a weight. I started to feel defeated, and on several occasions, I picked up the phone to call and back out but something within would not let me. I felt on edge and overwhelmed. I prayed and asked God, why? If it was to make me stronger, was I not strong enough? Had I not gone through enough already? How much more did I need to go through? How many more challenges did I need? After questioning and crying out, I would get up, ask Him to forgive my moment of despair and move forward.

The baccalaureate was approaching. I had to concentrate on finishing my speech. I struggled with what I would tell these students, struggling myself with uncertainty and sometimes feeling defeated. I finally came up with a theme: "Never Give Up on You." I combined my theme with the senior class' theme selected from Walt Disney, "All of our dreams can come true if we have the courage to pursue." Courage was something I was definitely struggling with. I told myself, *if we don't find an attorney, I will represent the case myself.* Seriously, I did not want it to come down to this.

We found a good deal on Robyn's prom dress. We took photos sending them to family and friends. In the early days of her rehabilitation, we were told she would never get to this point.

The young man that was going to escort her to the prom backed out at the last minute. Her brother came home just in time to be her escort. Although he was not her ideal date, she made her prom. The next weekend was the Baccalaureate. That Sunday morning, I sent the kids to church. I needed a moment of silence and time alone. I prayed and praised God and asked him to please help me through this and give these young people something to take with them along life's journey.

Although I was nervous, I was glad I had the opportunity to share with them the goodness of God. I fought back tears as I told them of Robyn's journey, from brain-dead to her 2012 graduation. I stressed to them the importance of perseverance and courage. I had my 15-year-old record with my phone. I have yet mustered the courage to view it. I think just knowing I lived through it is enough.

The following week was graduation. My niece called from California and asked if she could come. She wanted to stay with us. I told her, "the more the merrier. It may be a little cramped in my apartment, but we're all family, so c'mon."

I rose early the morning of graduation. I praised God and attempted to get all my tears out that morning. It was a long journey. We had no clue how we were going to make it to this day. When I brought Robyn home in February of 2008, I was overwhelmed with the idea of caring for her and her brothers. I did not believe I could do it. My mom stayed a total of eight months with me and when she left I was scared.

Robyn still needed a lot of care. I could not work. I tried to get financial support but as a parent, the state would not assist me to care for Robyn, but would pay strangers to do it. I tried outside help for a short time, but it did not work.

Although the feeding tube and tracheotomy had been removed before leaving the hospital, Robyn still required a lot of care. It was like bringing home a newborn at 13-years-old. She could not walk. She still needed some assistance with eating. She could not dress herself or bathe herself. She needed assistance with all of her personal needs.

The nurses and therapists at Primary Children's Hospital in Salt Lake City, Utah, trained me well. I learned how to transfer Robyn in and out of her wheelchair. I was taught how to bathe her using a shower chair. I was also trained on the feeding tube and the tracheotomy. Even though I was not confident that I could care for her at home, I prayed, and God gave me the strength to do it.

I could not work and care for Robyn. I resigned from my job which was a major financial blow. We eventually moved from our home with more than 3000 square feet into an apartment with less than 1200. I was actually excited because it relieved me of the stress of making the monthly note. We made it with the help of family, friends, church family, and most importantly, by the grace of God.

May 29, 2012, graduation day. We made it! As I watched her excitement, I felt a sense of calm, like everything was going to be alright. When Robyn's name was called during the ceremony, her class gave her a standing ovation. As a matter of fact, everyone in the gym was standing. She walked across the stage with an urgency. When the school official reached for her hand, she nearly pulled him over trying to hug him. She was so funny! So excited! So alive!

Following graduation, the seniors had the traditional all night party for the graduates. I committed myself to participate as a chaperon. This was before Mr. Nalder informed me that he was withdrawing from the case. Consequently, the court hearing was scheduled for the day after graduation. Since I had family members visiting, I asked them to attend with me.

The next morning, May 30, 2012, we attended Mr. Nalder's hearing to petition the court to withdraw from the case. I did not have to appear, but I wanted to hear Mr. Nalder's argument for requesting to withdraw from the case. Well, to my surprise he did not have to present an argument, as the court document stated he would. When the judge asked me if I objected, I responded, "No, because Mr. Nalder and Dr. Garland had falsified Robyn's medical records. I want to request a continuance so that I can press criminal charges." The judge said that I could not request a continuance and that I had twenty more days to obtain counsel, represent myself or dismiss with prejudice. Mr. Nalder asked the judge to be excused. He nearly ran out of the courtroom. As I have no knowledge of court proceedings, I just turned and walked away. My sister grabbed me and said "The judge hasn't dismissed us yet."

"Oh," I said. Then stopped and waited for the judge to dismiss.

——— ✧ ———

"Mom," Robyn brought me out of my muse.

"Yeah,"

"Love ya. See you later," Robyn replied as she exited the car.

After I dropped Robyn off, I drove to Target and pulled into the lot. I usually waited there until the library opened. I could not afford to drive back to San Gabriel.

I decided to open the letter. Not surprising, Judge Tingey did not acknowledge our request to turn the case over for a criminal investigation. He did grant our request to dismiss without prejudice. Dismissing without prejudice means she can refile at another time.

Chapter 6

Corruption Among Idaho Falls Officials

[1] ...Beware ye of the leaven of the Pharisees, which is hypocrisy.
[2] For there is nothing covered, that shall not be revealed; neither hid, that shall not be known.

[3] Therefore whatsoever ye have spoken in darkness shall be heard in the light; and that which ye have spoken in the ear in closets shall be proclaimed upon the housetops.

Luke 12: 1-3 (KJV).

It was about the end of April or beginning of May 2012, when I first visited the Idaho Falls Police Department. At that time, I was troubled by Mr. Nalder and Mr. Barton's attempts to intimidate me with fraudulent information. I was unsure where to seek help from but felt the police department was the most likely place. Mr. Nalder and Barton had not only participated in undermining Robyn's malpractice case, but my thoughts were, they had to have crossed a criminal code in their attempts to coerce me to dismiss the civil case with prejudice.

My only interaction with the Idaho Falls Police before this time were two traffic violations several years ago. I had heard negative comments about the Idaho Falls Police Department. Like other cities, the police did not have a good reputation in the minority community, but I did not let this stop me from filing a complaint. I decided to take a friend with me to file the criminal complaint.

When we entered the station, an older gentleman was seated at the reception desk. I informed him I wanted to file a complaint. He gave me a form to fill out. I remember thinking this is not going to be large enough. I took the half sheet of paper and listed my complaint against Dr. Garland, Mr. Nalder and Mr. Barton. I also listed the Idaho codes they violated (18:2601 and 2602). I also filed a complaint against Mr. Nalder and Mr. Barton for conspiracy. I returned the form to the older man. He asked us to take a seat and an officer would be out to speak with us.

My friend and I waited so long, I jokingly said, "they must be performing a background check on me for filing a complaint against those three." Officer Deedee, a bald, white gentleman, came out and spoke with us. He appeared sympathetic to my concerns, but he did not take a report. He informed my friend and me that he had never had a complaint of this nature and had no knowledge on how to write a report on it. According to him, if he took a report, he had no idea who to send it to because the police did not handle these matters.

My friend and I listened to him. We knew he was lying but was not sure what to do next. So, we left. That evening when I drove up to my apartment, before getting out of the car, I called the Idaho Attorney General's Office. A lady answered the phone. I explained my complaint and the policeman's refusal to take a report. She informed me that the complaint needed to be sent to the Bonneville County Prosecutor. He handled this type of complaint. She also said it was strange for the policeman not to take the report and forward it on to the prosecutor. She also informed me to make sure I knew what Idaho codes were violated before returning.

A couple of days later, Robyn and I visited the police department. I asked for Officer Deedee. I explained to the older gentleman behind the desk that I had spoken with Officer Deedee before. The older man remembered me. He asked me to take a seat. He informed Officer Deedee that I was out front. Robyn and I waited a long while before Officer Deedee came out.

This time Deedee's demeanor was rude and abrupt. I informed him that I had spoken with the Idaho Attorney General's Office and was told he should have taken the report and passed it on to the county prosecutor. He then replied that I was just upset because Mr. Nalder withdrew from the case and that he was instructed by his superior not to take a report. I asked to speak with his superior.

Deedee left and returned with an officer from internal affairs. Deedee's superior had already left for the day. I was told by the internal affairs officer that it was not necessary to visit the station again and to call before returning. I began calling the next Monday. I left messages for Deedee's superior. He also refused to take a report. From there I spoke with Lieutenant Cook and then Captain McBride. They too refused to take a written report.

On June 1, 2012, I visited the police station again. This time I filled out separate complaints on Mr. Nalder, Mr. Barton and Garland. I wanted to make sure I had followed directions. Initially I used one form for all of them. While I was there, I also asked where the Bonneville County Prosecutor's office was located. I found out it was down the hall from the front desk. I walked down and asked to speak with someone regarding my complaint. I was told by a young lady in the office that my complaint had to come through the police and they could not help me. I eventually made an appointment to meet with Police Chief Roos on June 8, 2012.

In the meantime, the hearing was scheduled for May 30, 2012, before Judge Tingey on Mr. Nalder's request to withdraw from the medical malpractice case. Mr. Nalder was supposed to give an argument before the court regarding his reasoning for withdrawing. I attended only to see if he would lie before the court as he did to Robyn's father and me. Also in attendance at the hearing were Robyn, my sister, my niece, and my two sons.

As I had no knowledge of court proceedings before this time, I was not expecting Judge Tingey to ask me if I objected to Nalder withdrawing, or the consequences to my answer. When he asked if I had any objections, I replied, "No, because I believed Mr. Nalder and Mr. Barton had conspired with Dr. Garland in falsifying Robyn's medical records." I also asked for a continuance on the case while criminal charges were filed. Mr. Nalder and I were sitting side by side before Judge Tingey. I noticed Nalder never raised his head while I was speaking, but started writing something down on a tablet.

Judge Tingey denied my request and granted Nalder's request for withdrawal without an argument from Mr. Nalder. This saved Mr. Nalder from perjuring himself before the court. Mr.

Nalder asked Judge Tingey if he could leave before court was dismissed, and his request was granted. He almost ran out of the courtroom. It would have been funny, but I figured he probably left to notify others of my plans to seek criminal charges against the trio (Garland, Nalder and Barton). While Judge Tingey's denial for time to seek criminal charges concerned me, I was not discouraged because I planned to continue to seek redress through the filing of a criminal report with the Idaho Falls Police Department.

When Robyn and I met with Chief Roos of the Idaho Falls Police department it was obvious that the meeting was just to appease me. I produced Robyn's medical records and a copy of Idaho Statutes 18:2601-2602. I could tell he was not expecting to have this conversation with me. He and I debated the validity of the statutes as they related to Dr. Garland's fraudulent actions during the civil court proceedings. Finally, when his placating did not work, he called in a Deputy Attorney from the Bonneville Prosecutor's office (Jay), and they attempted to dissuade me. They too refused to take a written report of my complaint.

Jay informed me that Idaho Statute 18-2601 and 2602 did not apply in the case against Dr. Garland. Not because the doctor did not do wrong, but because I did not know whether or not he intended to use the false information. Yet, the statute also stated that allowing fraudulent information to be used during a court/trial or investigation was a felony. So regardless of Dr. Garland's intent, he falsified the medical records. He knew they were false, yet, allowed them to be introduced during a civil trial/court case as factual.

Chief Roos, assured me that he was sure Dr. Garland was sorry, and that there was nothing legally they could do. I informed Roos and Jay that I knew who I was up against, but that I was not going to give up because I knew a criminal law had been broken as well as civil rights violated. If the police were not going to help, I still needed to find an attorney for Robyn. Judge Tingey had given me twenty days to find an attorney, represent the case myself or dismiss with prejudice.

I called on many attorneys, but none of them would take the case after I explained what they were up against. Some commented off the record. One attorney told me that if I took the case on myself, the defendant's side and the court would wait me out. They would wait for me to miss a court date or not respond, and then dismiss the case. As I look back, I see some instances of this.

On July 10, 2012, I had a court date. I took two friends with me to the session. We waited in the courtroom for about 30 minutes past the appointed time. The court clerk happened to pass through and saw us. She asked why we were there. I told her I was scheduled to appear before Judge Tingey. She went to the back to speak with the judge. She came back and stated that it had been canceled by Judge Tingey. Yet, I did not receive a letter regarding the cancellation. She asked me to come to her desk. I followed her back to her desk. Judge Tingey's door was opened, but he did not look up at me. She rescheduled the court date. I wondered if this is what that attorney was referring to when he said they would wait me out. I often ponder what would have happened had I not shown up. Would the case have been dismissed with prejudice for my failure to show up in court?

I was also told by the court that the trial date would be discontinued to allow time to find another attorney. Yet, it was never changed. Some of the lawyers I contacted informed me that the trial date was still set for October 23, 2012. When I called and asked the court clerk about it, she said that she had no idea why the system had not updated because she made the changes. I am not sure if this made a big difference in attorneys taking the case on, or if it was some kind of signal to avert them. I also recognized that with Attorney Nalder lying to prospective attorneys, there was no way that we would retain one.

One attorney informed me that it was impossible to get a negligence verdict in Idaho Falls, without a doctor in the area to verify the medical standard of care. He stated that Idaho Falls was one of the most conservative areas in the US and that was the problem that I was running into. He referred me to another attorney. The attorney he referred me to knew Mr. Barton and would not consider taking on the case. I realize now that Mr. Barton was probably brought aboard not to help the case, but because of his standing in the legal community in Idaho, to deter others from taking on the case. It appeared that many of the attorneys I spoke with had knowledge of Mr. Barton not Mr. Nalder.

In my search, I came across an older attorney who did not seem at all moved by what I was up against. He could not take on our case because he had just taken on a case against a large employer in the area. I informed him of the intent of Mr. Nalder to defraud the case. He and I talked about the lack of integrity in the legal system in Idaho. He said it was unfortunate and asked if I had considered Breck Barton. I informed him that Mr. Barton was a part of the deceptive plot to undermine Robyn's malpractice lawsuit. He referred me to several attorneys, but none would take on the case.

June 10, the same date of the hearing, I left Idaho Falls to take Robyn and her brother to Memphis, Tennessee to spend a month with their father and other family. I was so disturbed by the court proceeding, that when I helped Robyn in the car, I placed a file folder of court information on top of the car and forgot it. As we entered Interstate 15, I heard a thump, but when I looked out my rear view mirror I saw nothing behind me. I suddenly remembered I left the file folder on top of the SUV. I pulled over and the only item I found was my book on "How to Represent Yourself in Court." I turned around and headed back to where I entered the interstate. Sure enough, my file folder was in the center lane. Someone had run over it. My documents were spread out all over the interstate and the center median.

"Mom you are not gonna stop and get those papers, are you?" My son said.

My first thought was to leave them, but there were documents that I needed for the case. I pulled over and told Robyn and her brother to stay in the SUV. I started collecting documents that were spread out for at least half a mile. My son eventually got out and started helping me collect them. It was good that it was early and there was very little traffic, or I would have left them there. After collecting them and starting back, we realized ants were on some of the documents. I pulled over again, shook the documents off and placed them in a plastic bag and then got back on the interstate.

The trip to Memphis took two days. When we stopped in the evenings I was too wound up to sleep. I started reading through the book and learning legal jargon. When we made it to Memphis, I did not want to return to Idaho, but my older son was there and I had not emptied the apartment. I returned to Idaho. While I was away, I received a letter from Robyn's program. The start date had changed, and we needed to be in California a week earlier.

I was still trying to figure out how we were going to make the original date, so the change certainly threw me off balance. I told my son to give his notice at his job and I gave mine. We packed up the apartment, gave away a lot of items, and threw out a lot of stuff. When we pulled out of Idaho for the final time, I felt a burden lifted. I had no idea how to fight the case from California, but I knew I was ready to leave Idaho.

Although, I eventually took on the case myself, I continued to search for an attorney to represent Robyn's interest. After I was removed, because Nalder failed to file my claim in the case, I continued to help Robyn fight it herself. Of course, we eventually filed to have it dismissed without prejudice and asked for it to be turned over for a criminal investigation, again. And again, Judge Tingey did not address our request for a criminal investigation but granted a dismissal without prejudice in October of 2012.

At this time, we were struggling to find a place to live in California. I decided to wait until I heard from the Idaho Bar Association before contacting anyone else in Idaho regarding the case. We stayed with a relative as long as we could, but soon found ourselves homeless. I considered returning to Memphis, but my children wanted to stay in California. My children encouraged me and believed we would find a place. We lived in the Comfort Inn for about two months and before that the Howard Johnson Hotel. An organization that assist homeless families, Illumination Foundation, helped us find temporary accommodations, but it was not functional for Robyn, and my older son could not live there with us. We continued to live at the Comfort Inn and my mom helped with the payment for the room.

With help from our church family in California, my older son eventually found a job. The Illumination foundation and my mom helped us with a down payment on an apartment, and we moved in a few days before Christmas of 2012. It was a struggle and many times I wanted to turn back. I never would have imagined that my children would be encouraging me to not give up, but they did, and I am glad for their determined spirits.

The Lord showed me again how wonderful He is. Christmas of 2012, our church family showered us with gifts and helped to furnish our apartment. They even brought my son a violin when they found out he played the violin. He performed Silent Night at the Christmas Eve service. While we had a lot of challenges, we have had a lot of people to bless us and love us through the struggle. I think God intentionally placed me at a predominantly white church while I was fighting predominantly white people in Idaho because it kept me mentally balanced in my thinking.

January of 2013, I collected my mail from the San Gabriel, California address I initially had it forwarded to. I had a letter from the Idaho Bar Association. According to the Bar Association, they found no grounds for my complaint against Mr. Nalder. Before I received the letter, I was in the process of constructing a letter to the Governor of Idaho, Idaho Falls Representatives, and City Council. I put off writing my letter to the Idaho Officials and responded to the Bar.

Of course, the Bar scheduled a hearing in response to my letter and later found no grounds for my appeal. I decided to return to the police because I knew laws had been violated regarding defrauding a court process. Well, at this time Mayor Fuhriman was in the process of stepping down because of an illness. Police Chief Roos was no longer there, and Captain McBride was now Chief of Police.

I first wrote the Mayor of Idaho Falls asking for his assistance in getting the police to enforce Idaho Statute 18:2601 and 2602.

TITLE 18 -CRIMES AND PUNISHMENTS CHAPTER 26-EVIDENCE FALSIFIED OR CONCEALED AND WITNESSES INTIMIDATED OR BRIBED-18-2601. FALSIFYING EVIDENCE -- OFFERING FORGED OR FRAUDULENT DOCUMENTS IN EVIDENCE. Every person who, upon any trial, proceeding, inquiry or investigation whatever authorized or permitted by law, offers in evidence as genuine or true, any book, paper, document, record, or other instrument in writing, knowing the same to have been forged or fraudulently altered or antedated, is guilty of felony.

> *18-2602. PREPARING FALSE EVIDENCE. Every person guilty of preparing any false or antedated book, paper, record, instrument in writing, or other matter or thing, with intent to produce it, or allow it to be produced, for any fraudulent or deceitful purpose, as genuine or true, upon any trial, proceeding or inquiry whatever, authorized by law, is guilty of felony .*

Robyn and I both sent letters to Mayor Fuhriman. He replied that he had to consult the City Attorney before making a decision. I had no confidence that he would support us, but Robyn had confidence in him. So, I decided to be silent. Robyn and her aide spent half a school day in 2012 with Mayor Fuhriman as part of Disability Rights Day. She was impressed with his participation in the community and his declaration of concern for all of the citizens in Idaho Falls. Robyn's letter dated April 23, 2013:

> *Dear Mayor Fuhriman,*
>
> *It is me, Robyn Edwards. I participate in the Disability Rights Mentoring Day in 2012 and selected to spend the day with you. I was really moved by your love for the people in Idaho Falls.*
>
> *I am writing because I am seeking justice. Last year, I found out that Dr. Erich Garland changed my medical records the day of my stroke. He added migraine headaches to my files. I never had migraine headaches. My mom said he even stated that I had some that lasted all day. I cannot believe he did this.*
>
> *There is no way my Mom could have told him I had headaches with the numbness I experienced because I did not have headaches, only numbness in my limbs. I know people make mistakes, but Dr. Garland needs to own up to his negligence and not continue to cover it up.*
>
> *He destroyed my dreams. I had plans of running in the Olympics and attending Yale University. I had just been inducted into the honor society the spring before my stroke.*

I felt like I was at the peak of my life and in seconds everything was gone. I lost my friends.

In May of last year my Mom and I visited the Idaho Falls Police Department 3 times to file a police report on Dr. Garland for falsifying my medical records. We were turn away and no one would take the report.

I am writing because I want an official police report filed against Dr. Erich Garland for falsifying my medical records. I pray that you will help us.

Sincerely,
Robyn Edwards

Although I had serious reservations about Mayor Fuhriman, I would not allow my knowledge of him to interfere with how Robyn felt about him. We mailed the letter along with the one I wrote. I had also started a petition online asking citizens to get involved and petition for Mayor Fuhriman to step in and force the police to uphold the Idaho statute.

Incidentally, I met Mayor Fuhriman when I was an active member of the African American Alliance (AAA) in Idaho Falls. In 2011, I was asked by the AAA president to apply for an open position one of the AAA members vacated on the Mayor's Race Relations' Committee. Well, at this time I also had the complaint in against an employer in Idaho Falls for EEO violations.

I met with Mayor Fuhriman because I wanted to introduce myself before I submitted my application for the position on the committee. I also mentioned my complaint and the difficulties minorities in the community have with this employer. During the meeting he did not say much. I imagine I was foreign to him, a female, black at that, daring to confront the inhumane practices in the Idaho Falls community. The mayor's secretary contacted me weeks later to inform me that Mayor Fuhriman and another committee member decided not to fill the open position.

Well, the Mayor asked for the city attorney to make a recommendation on whether to get involved. Remember, we were only asking that the police investigate the violation of an Idaho

Statute. In a letter dated June 6, 2013, Mayor Fuhriman sent his regrets that the city would not take any action based on information City Attorney Randy Fife provided.

In the letter City Attorney Fife wrote on May 23, 2013, addressed to the mayor, he provided several untrue statements. First of all, he stated that I had contacted the Idaho Medical Board, which I had not at this time. Second, he stated that the police properly followed up on the police report filed by me. I have emails that show that a report was not taken until after Attorney Fife's letter was written. The police never took a report in 2012 and refused to even look at the information I provided, and certainly did not ask for any copies of the documents to review. It would be interesting to know where Mr. Fife and Prosecutor Bruce Pickett obtained information about the case to make a decision. Please read the emails from the Idaho Falls Police department at the end of this chapter.

Mr. Fife also mentions that the legal system decided that it did not appear that the prosecution of Dr. Garland under Code 18-2602 would be "proper." Not sure if it is necessary for it to be proper, I would think if he violated a "legal" code, the "legal" action to take would be to prosecute him. When is it "proper" to prosecute someone, and under what discriminating factors does the Idaho Falls police and Attorney Pickett prosecute people for felony offenses?

In the next sentence Fife mentions the Idaho Board of Medicine again, "Apparently, the Idaho Board of Medicine has not disciplined him." I thought this was an interesting declaration, especially, since I had not contacted them yet. I also thought maybe he made the statement because he knew how they would rule before we filed. I have attached the letter from the Idaho Board of Medicine which verifies when they received my complaint against Garland.

He goes on to mention the ruling of the Idaho Bar Association and that he had spoken with one of the attorneys I filed a complaint against. Well, I think it is obvious now that the Idaho Bar Association did not investigate my complaint either. If any of them had called and verified the expert's statements, they would have found out that Mr. Nalder and Mr. Barton lied about the expert changing his testimony.

As for the Attorney General's office, which Mr. Fife also mentions in the letter, I requested assistance from that office when the Idaho Falls police refused to take a report and investigate. They responded that their abilities to intervene in matters of local government and judiciary are limited. That letter is also attached.

While, I am astonished by all the lies, I am even more stunned by their willingness to place them in writing. This proves to me how bold they are and how dangerous they are to the general public. Not to mention the elected officials and public servants who are supposed to protect the interests of "all" of the citizens. Mr. Fife obviously lied to Mayor Fuhriman. The police never took a report, and the only information reviewed was what I sent to Mayor Fuhriman. The information that the police refused to take from me last year was submitted to the police after Mr. Fife wrote his letter. Consequently, a report was finally taken by the police, but it was after I contacted the Idaho Falls City Council. Mayor Fuhriman's response, Attorney Fife's letter, and the response from the Idaho Attorney General's Office follow this page. Also, the letter acknowledging the Idaho Medical Board's receipt of Robyn's complaint follows.

CITY OF IDAHO FALLS

Office of the Mayor
City Hall
Idaho Falls, Idaho 83405

Jared Fuhriman
Mayor

June 6, 2013

Veverly Edwards

Re: April 23, 2013 Letter

Dear Ms. Edwards:

I received your letter of April 23, 2013, and its materials several weeks ago. I asked the City Attorney, Randy Fife, to review those materials, and to make recommendations regarding them.

Attached is a copy of his May 23, 2013 Memorandum to me, for your review and information.

I spoke with Mr. Fife about his review, findings and recommendations, and agree with them. While I am very sympathetic to your situation, I do not feel that the City has failed in any duty or responsibility, or made incorrect decisions. For those reasons, the City will not be supporting your efforts to have Dr. Gardner prosecuted.

My best wishes to you and your family.

Sincerely,

Jared D. Fuhriman
Mayor of the City of Idaho Falls

JDF/co

Encl.: Memorandum
c: Robyn Edwards w/encl.

P. O. Box 50220 • 308 Constitution Way, Idaho Falls, Idaho 83405 • (208) 612-8235 • Fax (208) 612-8560

LEGAL DEPARTMENT

CITY OF IDAHO FALLS
RANDALL D. FIFE, CITY ATTORNEY
PO BOX 50220
IDAHO FALLS, IDAHO 83405
Telephone No.: (208) 612-8178
www.idahofallsidaho.gov

MEMORANDUM

DATE: May 23, 2013
TO: Mayor Jared D. Fuhriman
FROM: City Attorney, Randall D. Fife
RE: Review of Veverly Edwards' April 23, 2013 Materials

Dear Mayor:

I reviewed the materials sent by Ms. Veverly Edwards, which included:

1. A four (4) page letter;
2. An excerpt from a deposition dated September 22, 2011;
3. An eight (8) page letter dated March 22, 2012 from [redacted], M.D.; and
4. A three (3) page opinion letter from Jill Wilson dated April 18, 2013 (including Ms. Wilson's CV and selected medical records of Robyn Edwards).

The essence of Ms. Edwards' claim appears to be that Ms. Edwards' daughter, Robyn, sought medical treatment and subsequently experienced a stroke, which has left her disabled. Ms. Edwards sought the assistance of some local attorneys who later withdrew from representing her.

Subsequent to that, Ms. Edwards filed a complaint with the Idaho Falls Police Department claiming that Robyn's treating physician, Dr. Garland, falsified Robyn's medical records. Ms. Edwards filed a complaint against Dr. Garland with the Idaho State Board of Medicine. Ms. Edwards also filed a complaint with the Idaho State Bar against her former attorneys, Lance Nalder and Breck Barton.

Currently, it appears that Ms. Edwards is attempting to pursue redress for alleged injustices by sponsoring a website petition on *change.org* entitled "Disabled Teen Requests Equal Protection Under the Law – Mayor Fuhriman Please Enforce Idaho Statutes 18-2601 and 2602." The website petition includes a copy of the letter you received dated April 23, 2013.

Without going into detail, I reviewed the materials provided and have determined that the Police Department appropriately followed up on the Police Report filed by Ms. Edwards.

Memo to Mayor Fuhriman
Page 2
May 23, 2013

Based upon the information available to the Police Department, the legal system decided that it did not appear that prosecution of Dr. Garland under Idaho Code § 18-2602 would be proper. I confirmed that decision with Bonneville County Prosecutor, Bruce Pickett.

Apparently, the Idaho State Board of Medicine has not disciplined Dr. Garland.

One of the attorneys involved with Ms. Edwards, stated that the complaint made by Ms. Edwards to the Idaho State Bar did not result in a finding of wrongdoing against either Mr. Nalder or Mr. Barton.

I confirmed with the Idaho Attorney General's office that they are not pursuing any action against anyone at this time.

My review of the information provided by Ms. Edwards, coupled with my experience as an attorney involved in personal injury litigation, claims, and risk management, leaves me to conclude that, although Ms. Edwards and her daughter Robyn, have suffered a substantial loss, the Idaho Falls Police Department gave reasonable consideration relative to the police report made.

The City does not control, nor does it have jurisdiction over Dr. Garland, Mr. Nalder, Mr. Barton, the Bonneville County Prosecutor's Office, the Idaho Attorney General Office, the Idaho State Board of Medicine, or the Idaho State Bar. While I am sympathetic to their plight, I do not recommend that the City change the decisions that have been made by it, nor do I recommend proceeding beyond the efforts made by the City to date.

It is my impression that Ms. Edwards is very intelligent, able, motivated, and that she has pursued (and is pursuing) many avenues that may be able to bring her satisfaction. I wish her the best; however, I do not believe that the City has an active role at this time in such efforts.

Respectfully,

Randall D. Fife
City Attorney

RDF/co

STATE OF IDAHO

OFFICE OF THE ATTORNEY GENERAL

LAWRENCE G. WASDEN

May 29, 2012

Veverly M. Edwards
555 S Old Butte Highway #602
Idaho Falls, ID 83402

Dear Ms. Edwards:

Attorney General Wasden asked that I respond to your letter requesting to file criminal charges Dr. Erich Garland and attorney Lance Nalder.

Unfortunately, the ability of the Attorney General to intervene in matters of local government and the judiciary is strictly limited by statute and case law.

Members of the Attorney General's staff are assigned to assist prosecutors and law enforcement in the prosecution of criminal offenses. However, these requests must be made by the respective prosecutor who has statutory and common law jurisdiction over all actions, civil or criminal, in the district court of their county. Idaho Code § 31-2227 states, "[I]t is hereby declared to be the policy of the State of Idaho that the primary duty of enforcing all of the penal provisions of any and all statutes of this state, in any court, is vested in the sheriff and prosecuting attorney of each of the several counties."

The Attorney General has no supervisory authority over local law enforcement agencies or private attorneys and cannot intervene in this matter.

I hope this letter is helpful to you in understanding the statutory limitations of this office and the reason we cannot provide the assistance you have requested.

Sincerely,

KRISS BIVENS CLOYD
Constituent Information Specialist

/kbc

P.O. Box 83720, Boise, Idaho 83720-0010
Telephone: (208) 334-2400, FAX: (208) 854-8071
Located at 700 W. Jefferson Street, Suite 210

STATE OF IDAHO
BOARD OF MEDICINE

1755 Westgate Dr., Ste 140
Boise, Idaho 83704
(208) 327-7000
FAX (208) 327-7005
E-Mail info@bom.idaho.gov
Website bom.idaho.com

September 9, 2013

CONFIDENTIAL

ROBYN O EDWARDS

Re: Complaint against Erich Wesley Garland MD

Dear Ms. Edwards:

During its meeting on September 6, 2013, the Idaho State Board of Medicine (Board) considered the results of the investigation into your complaint against Erich Wesley Garland MD.

After review of correspondence, medical records and information obtained during the investigation of this complaint, the Board determined that the facts do not warrant formal disciplinary action and acted to close consideration of the matter at this time.

Although formal action was not taken, in some instances informal, confidential, disciplinary action is initiated. In these cases, the Board directs attention to its concerns through education, training or other non-disciplinary means as an opportunity for the licensee to improve his/her practice.

Thank you for allowing the Board to review the information you provided regarding the professional practice and conduct of one of our licensees.

A record of this investigation will remain at the Board's office.

Sincerely,

Nancy M Kerr

Nancy Kerr
Executive Director
Idaho State Board of Medicine

NK/cp

What puzzled me most about City Attorney Fife's letter is his statement regarding it not being "proper" to prosecute Dr. Garland. I do not think Mr. Fife meant for the letter to be forwarded to me, but because Mayor Fuhriman was stepping down, I believe someone just copied the letter and sent it to me and stated that the Mayor was in agreement.

I intentionally blacked out the name of the expert witness on the letter because he was not a part of this deception. His name is in the files. The police and prosecuting attorney have access to his information.

I also wondered if the police and the City of Idaho Falls had a conflict of interest handling my complaint because of an initiative Dr. Garland headed that the City may have had interests in. I then reread the article in the Post Register's Spring/Summer magazine 2012. The article on stroke care at EIRMC in which the Joint Commission gave them the elite gold seal, was a concerted effort by many in the community. It appears that many doctors in Idaho Falls, the emergency room staff at EIRMC, paramedics and firefighters took part, and that Dr. Garland appeared to be the lead on the initiative. I think it is logical to say that if the firefighters and paramedics took part, the city had a stake in it too, but I could be wrong. This would probably shed light on the statements made by the prosecuting attorney and the city attorney on why it would not be "proper" to prosecute Dr. Garland

The article in the Post Register further stated that Eastern Idaho Regional Medical Center was the second hospital in Idaho to be verified as a Primary Stroke Center. Not sure what this meant on the state level. I am not sure what a conviction of falsifying medical records of a 13-year-old girl, after causing her to have a massive stroke and disabling her for life, would have on Dr. Garland's reputation, or this preventative stoke initiative. I could only assume from the actions of Dr. Garland, Mr. Nalder, Mr. Barton, the Mayor, the Idaho Falls City Attorney, Bonneville County Prosecutor, state level boards and all the other officials who did not respond, that the impact would have probably been negative and significant.

Mr. Fife, as with Attorney Nalder, has attempted to portray me as a mother whose child met with an unfortunate medical condition and blamed Dr. Garland. The reality is Dr. Garland not only misdiagnosed, but he also prescribed the wrong drug to a 13-year-old girl and almost killed her. He then changed her medical records to reflect the condition the drug is meant to treat. Innocent people do not falsify medical records and then use them to defraud the patient and family during a medical malpractice lawsuit.

What is utterly amazing is the number of officials willing to take part in the deception. On May 29, 2013, I decided to write the members of the Idaho Falls City Council. The only response I received was from City Councilwoman Sharon Parry. If city councilwoman Parry had not responded, and requested the police's responsibility, a report would have never been taken. While the others have portrayed me as an individual who is falsely accusing Dr. Garland, I have patiently collected the information and lies they have told.

The most unsettling fact is that leaders in the Idaho Falls community have taken part in the fraudulent cover up: the Police Chief, Mayor, City Attorney, and Prosecuting Attorney, all taking part in the deceptive plot to undermine me. Again, what they fail to realize, and the truth I stand on, is that I am not the only one knowledgeable of the fact that Robyn never had migraine headaches. In their attempts to quiet my voice, God has shown me a way to expose it to the general public. These people are willing to sacrifice their positions, livelihoods and embarrass their families for Dr. Garland. I guess some might find this an admirable trait. I find it repulsive.

After writing the letter to Mayor Fuhriman, I contacted the police again. I first spoke to an officer who attempted to assure me that Chief Roos was correct in his decision the previous year. I told him I did not agree because Chief Roos and the deputy prosecutor attempted to convince me that I had to know Garland's intent and that if I could not determine his intent in falsifying the documents, there was no way to establish whether or not a crime had been committed.

I informed the officer that according to the statute concerning defrauding a court process, either intent needed to be established or the information had to have been used during the court process, which included the investigative part of the process. When the officer could not convince me that nothing criminal transpired, I was referred to his superior. His superior tried to convince me that the statute of limitations had run out because Dr. Garland had committed this offense in October of 2007. My question to this officer was, "How can the statute of limitations run out on fraud before it is discovered?" The fact that Dr. Garland falsified Robyn's records in October of 2007, had no bearing on the fraud he committed by allowing them to be presented in a court of law in 2012, as factual information. When I got tired of dealing with the Idaho Falls Police, I then wrote letters to the Governor of Idaho, Idaho Falls Representatives, and the Idaho Falls City Council. The following letter was sent to every member of the Idaho Falls City Council including Sharon Parry on May 29, 2013:

Council Member Parry,

My name is Veverly Edwards. I once worked for the State of Idaho at Idaho Falls Labor Department. My daughter was stricken with an illness in October of 2007. At that time my colleagues rallied around us and extended their love, concern, and support for my family. We really appreciated all that was done.

Today I am writing because I need assistance with another issue. After nearly losing my child in 2007, I found out that Dr. Eric Garland, a neurologist in Idaho Falls, Idaho gave Robyn a prescription drug (Zomig) that caused the massive stroke. Once he realized his grave error, he then changed her medical records to reflect migraine headache symptoms that she did not have. The drug, Zomig, is only given to treat migraine headaches. Robyn was having numbness in her limbs. She never had a migraine headache.

You are probably asking, why am I writing you instead of filing a Malpractice Lawsuit? Actually, we did file in 2009. The case was scheduled to go to trial last October. Six months before going to trial, the attorney representing our interests, G. Lance Nalder, withdrew from the case. I would have dismissed at that point had it not been for the fact that Nalder attempted to intimidate me with false medical records. I informed Nalder and the opposing side during a deposition that the document in question presented as a part of Robyn's records was not in my handwriting. I have since had a forensic document examiner review the document Nalder said compromised my testimony and the document is in Dr. Garland's handwriting.

These individuals made a mockery of my daughter's medical malpractice case and of Idaho's civil litigation process. Idaho Statute 18-2601 and 2602, states that it is a felony offense to introduce false information into any trial or court proceeding in Idaho even the investigative process. I have attempted several times to file a complaint with the Idaho Falls Police Department and they have refused to take a report. I have even written Mayor Fuhriman for his assistance.

I spoke with Captain Cook of the Idaho Falls Police Department on May 23, 2013. I realized after speaking with him he was just patronizing me. It ended with him stating that even if we could prove Dr. Garland falsified the records the statute of limitations had run out on Idaho 18: 2601-2602. He attempted to convince me that the time started when Garland falsified the records. However, it did not become a criminal offense until Dr. Garland used the documents during the court/trial process, so how could the statute of limitations for this offense start before he introduced and defrauded the court process? My belief is either the police cannot read and interpret the laws or they think the citizens are unread.

I would think that the representatives of the people of Idaho Falls would have a problem with this. It is a dangerous precedence to allow a doctor to blatantly and willfully falsify information, allow it to be used during a civil court proceeding, and not hold him accountable according to the statutes that cover such criminal behavior. This doctor's actions forever changed the life of a 13-year-old girl. Innocent people do not change records and defraud civil cases. We need help in getting a police report taken and an investigation in this doctor's criminal offense.

Sincerely
Robyn Edwards
Veverly Edwards

I was surprised and thankful for the immediate response from council member Parry:

Chief McBride:
Could you give me an opinion on the following email in regard to what the city police responsibility is and is not? I assume the other council members were sent this also, so you may want to consider sending a response to the full council.
FYI: Other than a general response from you as to what reports can or should be filed through our police department and as to what role the police have in filing such reports, I probably need to stay out of this one; there is a likely conflict of interest with the medical doctor named in this email.
Thank you,
Sharon Parry

After Council Member Parry's inquiry, the police finally contacted me regarding taking a report of my complaint. On June 4, 2013 Joe Crawley, Captain of the Detective Division of the Idaho Falls Police Department, emailed me regarding taking a police report. However, according to City Attorney Fife's letter, a report had already been taken. It is interesting that City Attorney Fife mentioned that he and Prosecuting Attorney Pickett reviewed information regarding my initial complaint, and based on the information available to the police, concluded that it was improper to prosecute Dr. Garland.

Consequently, the police refused to take the documentation that I presented to them in 2012 regarding my initial complaint. If they had this information, Captain Cawley of the Idaho Falls Police would not have emailed me requesting the information. Captain Cawley's email is below:

Ms. Edwards, my name is Joe Cawley and I am the Captain of the Detective Division for the *Idaho Falls Police Department. I have reviewed your latest inquiry with Chief McBride, Captain Cook and our County Prosecuting Attorney Bruce Pickett.*
There are several specific questions that we need answers to in order to determine if a criminal act has occurred, and if there is enough facts to warrant a criminal investigation.

The following questions are for you, and please include any supporting documentation that may help us make this determination.
1. Was the document(s) in question (the alleged forged notes) entered into evidence in a court proceeding?
2. If this document was submitted, when and who submitted it?
3. What is the name and credentials of the document or handwriting examiner used?
4. What is the status of the lawsuit, if any?
5. What evidence do you have that the notes have been forged?

These preliminary questions must be answered prior to opening a criminal investigation. As you know, time is of the essence due to possible statute of limitation issues.

I have written you instead of making a phone call for two reasons. One, I know you have talked with several people regarding this issue, and I don't want you to feel you have to "start from scratch" with me. The other reason is that I will need documentation regarding these questions, and a written request is easier to refer to than a telephone conversation. If you have any questions or concerns, please feel free to contact me either by phone or email.

Respectfully

Captain Joe Cawley

Detective Division
Idaho Falls Police Department

I sent him a response on June 5, 2013, informing him that I would need more time to collect the information for his response. He agreed, and on June 10, 2013 I emailed him my response:

Mr. Crawley,

My responses are below and I have attached documents to this email. I cannot attach the docs to one email. So I will send another with another set of documents
Responses to Forgery investigation:

1. *Was the document(s) in question (the alleged forged notes) entered into evidence in a court proceeding?*
   a. *One of the documents was used during my deposition (I will send the page of the deposition and the doc). This was the document that G. Lance Nalder informed my ex-husband and I that weakened/compromised my testimony and one of the reasons he withdrew.*
   b. *The expert witness was given these documents to review to make his testimony to the court. He even identified the inconsistencies in Dr. Garland's reports.*
   c. *On July 25, 2012 I submitted to court and plaintiff a set of responses to requests for admissions and production of documents. Question 15 asked "Please produce any and all records, documents and evidence of any kind which supports your contention that any medical records in this case were altered, falsified or changed in any way? I presented the documents that Dr. Garland altered. I am attaching the documents that were filed in court.*
2. *If this document was submitted, when and who submitted it?*
   My deposition was done September of 2011.

Dr. XXX, the expert witness testimony was filed with the court April 16, 2012 it was submitted by G. Lance Nalder

Veverly Edwards submitted response to question 15 above and documents requested to the court on July 25, 2012.

3. *What is the name and credentials of the document or handwriting examiner used?*

Jill Wilson-I am attaching her opinion and her resume is included

4. *What is the status of the lawsuit, if any?*

Robyn's interests were dismissed without prejudice

5. *What evidence do you have that the notes have been forged?*

If a doctor writes a history of a medical condition into a patient's file there should be evidence that this happened in the past. Well, there is no evidence because Robyn never had migraine headaches. There is a registration document that I did fill out during Robyn's visit to Dr. Garland that asked for past medical history. I did not check anything on the list (a copy is included). Headaches/migraine was the first condition. I am an educated person and I know how to fill out a form. If I did not check it on my form, where would Dr. Garland come up with a history of this condition?

There is also a school form in the stack of court documents. Dr. Garland told me and Robyn that she had a rare form of migraine that caused numbness (Hemiplegic), not headaches. I told the school nurse what he told me and she wrote it on the document. She filled the top part of the document out the day of Robyn's appointment with Garland because I went back to the school to inform her of what he told us. I signed the next day because I had to get something in writing that stated he had instructed her on how to take the medication. There is also a note that is included that was attached to this form. You are not supposed to give Zomig for Hemiplegic migraines, which she did not have that condition either.

Robyn has been seen by a doctor at least once every year since birth, there is no history of migraine headaches in her medical file. Not one registration document in Dr. Garland's files with my handwriting on it suggests she even had a headache certainly not migraine headaches. He only saw her once. Her referral was for numbness in her limbs. Robyn had a numbing sensation while we were there not a headache. Robyn is competent and can speak for herself. Her short term memory was affected by the stroke. Robyn had been seeing Dr. Moore at Idaho Falls Pediatrics for a several years. Dr. Moore or Porter has never seen her for a migraine headache. I am still going through the files to find her medical records prior to seeing Garland. I have them, just have a lot of boxes to go through. I could sign for you all to get copies from Idaho Falls Pediatrics.

She has other family members that lived with her (two brothers) if these headaches lasted all day, I would think it would be noticeable to others because it would have affected her ability to perform and attend activities and school. She has never been out of school for a headache. She was a very active student as well as other activities in the community. The school nurse at Eagle Rock Jr. High can testify to the fact that Robyn was not having migraine headaches because I spoke with her about Dr. Garland diagnosis her with a rare form of migraine that caused numbness instead of headaches. She should be able to testify to this because she knew Robyn. I have forgotten her name but I am sure the school district has records of who was assigned to Eagle Rock in October of 2007.

While I have attempted several times to get this address, I feel that someone in the police department has alliances or affiliations with this doctor and do not want him to be charged. I would never lie or attempt to destroy another person's character or reputation. Dr. Erich Garland falsified my child's medical records and then he and his attorney used them to make a mockery of Robyn's civil case against him.

Sincerely,
Veverly Edwards

On June 21, 2013, I spoke with and submitted an inquiry to the intake department of an attorney in Texas. I informed the person taking the intake information about the Police investigation into Dr. Garland's fraudulent acts during the civil court process. I was asked for a case number so that they could verify my comments. I told the person taking the information I was not given one.

After speaking with the Texas attorney's office, I wrote Captain Cawley of the Idaho Falls Police department requesting a case number. He informed me that he did not receive the attachments that I sent on June 10, 2013 and so a case number had not been assigned, yet. He needed the additional information to see if a criminal case was warranted. So, I forwarded the information again.

According to an email from Captain Cawley on July 22, 2013, the investigation was turned into the Bonneville Prosecuting Attorney on July 9, 2013. Cawley was awaiting the prosecutor's determination on how to proceed and would contact me as soon as he heard. The dates get confusing because when I spoke with him on June 21, he did not have enough information, yet, he sent the information on to the prosecuting attorney after stating that he did not have the necessary documentation. I am not surprised because the Idaho Falls Police have not given me any reason to believe they actually investigated. I again asked for a case number to reference my complaint. He said one still had not been assigned.

July 31, 2013, I received an email for Captain Cawley:

> *Ms. Edwards, the Prosecuting Attorney does not feel he has enough information for criminal prosecution at this time. I have assigned your case to Detective Steve Barnes. Detective Barnes has worked forgery and fraud cases for many years. He will be contacting you to obtain any further information he needs. He will also give you a case number. I will work with him and provide assistance as necessary.*

That same day I received an email from Detective Barnes:

> *Ms. Ververly Edwards,*
> *I have been assigned the case you have requested and am in the process of doing an investigation. If you could call me I*

would appreciate it. I need to get some personal information from you to make the report.
I also have a couple of questions I would like to ask to assist my investigation. I am in and out of my office throughout the day, so if I am not in when you call, please leave me a message with your name and Number, and I will call you back at my earliest convenience.

Sincerely,

Detective Steve Barnes
Idaho Falls Police

I returned Detective Barnes' call and answered his questions. I heard from him again on August 19, and he informed me that because of a letter that existed in the medical records, dated October 1, 2007 they were closing the investigation. Supposedly, this was Garland's defense. I asked Officer Barnes if he had read through the letter carefully and matched up the dates with information in the file. He said he had, but as you remember from chapter 3, the MRI was mentioned in the letter. The MRI was not ordered until October 2, 2007 and was confirmed by Dr. Garland on October 3rd. My question to Officer Barnes, "How can this be a defense when it is obvious that the letter was not written on October 1, 2007?" According to him, he did not have this document in the file. I then asked, "How can you investigate if you have not requested the entire file from Dr. Garland?" I forwarded the information to him.

I also forwarded to Detective Barnes the names and addresses of my ex-husband and sister, whom I spoke with on the evening of October 1, 2007. They could verify that the MRI was not ordered on October 1, 2007, and that the letter written and used as a defense is in itself fraudulent. It is impossible to write a letter on October 1, 2007, and mail it with information in it containing events that occurred after October 1, 2007.

As of today, November 30, 2013, I have not heard from Detective Barnes, I sent him an email today, and will include his response if I receive it before publishing this book. I doubt that the Idaho Falls police have investigated my concerns, especially since the prosecutor and city attorney do not believe it is "proper" to prosecute Dr. Garland.

Every time I address the devastation of October 4, 2007, I feel like I am on a roller coaster ride, free falling, trying to brace myself until it stops, and it stops only to begin again.

I constantly ask myself, "how can it be so difficult to get help from authorities when people have blatantly committed, not only civil offenses, but criminal offenses too?" But I guess when the police department is corrupt, and the politicians depend on the lack of integrity of the police to undermine the citizens to promote their agendas, and the courts pretend they do not see the injustices, there is little chance the citizens' civil/constitutional rights will be protected.

The following pages are email communications with the Idaho Falls City Council and the Idaho Falls Police Department.

Gmail

The Idaho Falls Police refuse to take a report and investigate

[redacted]@gmail.com [redacted]@gmail.com> Wed, May 29, 2013 at 1:00 PM
To: [redacted]@cableone.net

Council Member Parry,

My name is Veverly Edwards. I once worked for the State of Idaho at Idaho Falls Labor Department. My daughter was stricken with an illness in October of 2007. At that time my colleagues rallied around us and extended their love, concern, and support for my family. We really appreciated all that was done.

Today I am writing because I need assistance with another issue. After nearly losing my child in 2007, I found out that Dr. Eric Garland, a neurologist in Idaho Falls, Idaho gave Robyn a prescription drug (Zomig) that caused the massive stroke. Once he realized his grave error, he then changed her medical records to reflect migraine headache symptoms that she did not have. The drug, Zomig, is only given to treat migraine headaches. Robyn was having numbness in her limbs. She never had a migraine headache.

You are probably asking, why am I writing you instead of filing a Malpractice Lawsuit? Actually, we did file in 2009. The case was scheduled to go to trial last October. Six months before going to trial, the attorney representing our interests, G. Lance Nalder, withdrew from the case. I would have dismissed at that point had it not been for the fact that Nalder attempted to intimidate me with false medical records. I informed Nalder and the opposing side during a deposition that the document in question presented as a part of Robyn's records was not in my handwriting. I have since had a forensic document examiner review the document Nalder said compromised my testimony and the document is in Dr. Garland's handwriting.

These individuals made a mockery of my daughter's medical malpractice case and of Idaho's civil litigation process. Idaho Statute 18-2601 and 2602, states that it is a felony offense to introduce false information into any trail or court proceeding in Idaho even the investigative process. I have attempted several times to file a complaint with the Idaho Falls Police Department and they have refused to take a report. I have even written Mayor Fuhriman for his assistance.

I spoke with Captain Cook of the Idaho Falls Police Department on May 23, 2013. I realized after speaking with him he was just patronizing me. It ended with him stating that even if we could prove Dr. Garland falsified the records the statute of limitations had run out on Idaho 18: 2601-2602. He attempted to convince me that the time started when Garland falsified the records. However, it did not become a criminal offense until Dr. Garland used the documents during the court/trial process, so how could the statute of limitations for this offense start before he introduced and defrauded the court process? My belief is either the police cannot read and interpret the laws or they think the citizens are unread.

1/19/2014 Gmail - The Idaho Falls Police refuse to take a report and investigate

I would think that the representatives of the people of Idaho Falls would have a problem with this. It is a dangerous precedence to allow a doctor to blatantly and willfully falsify information, allow it to be used during a civil court proceeding, and not hold him accountable according to the statutes that cover such criminal behavior. This doctor's actions forever changed the life of a 13-year-old girl. Innocent people do not change records and defraud civil cases. We need help in getting a police report taken and an investigation in this doctor's criminal offense.

Sincerely

Robyn Edwards

Veverly Edwards

Sharon Parry [redacted]@cableone.net> Wed, May 29, 2013 at 3:31 PM
To: Mark McBride [redacted]@idahofallsidaho.gov>
Cc: [redacted]@gmail.com

Chief McBride:
Could you give me an opinion on the following email in regard to what the city police responsibility is and is not? I assume the other council members were sent this also, so you may want to consider sending a response to the full council.
FYI: Other than a general response from you as to what reports can or should be filed through our police department and as to what role the police have in filing such reports, I probably need to stay out of this one; there is a likely conflict of interest with the medical doctor named in this email.
Thank you,
Sharon Parry
[Quoted text hidden]

https://mail.google.com/mail/u/0/?ui=2&ik=201ecf8ea7&view=pt&search=inbox&th=13ef1e0b89c5078a 2/2

Gmail by Google

V. M. Edwards <[redacted]@gmail.com>

Forgery Investigation

6 messages

Joe Cawley [redacted]@idahofallsidaho.gov> Tue, Jun 4, 2013 at 2:54 PM
To: [redacted]@gmail.com" <[redacted]@gmail.com>
Cc: Mark McBride [redacted]@idahofallsidaho.gov>, Darren Cook [redacted]@idahofallsidaho.gov>

Ms. Edwards, my name is Joe Cawley and I am the Captain of the Detective Division for the Idaho Falls Police Department. I have reviewed your latest inquiry with Chief McBride, Captain Cook and our County Prosecuting Attorney Bruce Pickett.

There are several specific questions that we need answers to in order to determine if a criminal act has occurred, and if there is enough facts to warrant a criminal investigation.

The following questions are for you, and please include any supporting documentation that may help us make this determination.

1. Was the document(s) in question (the alleged forged notes) entered into evidence in a court proceeding?
2. If this document was submitted, when and who submitted it?
3. What is the name and credentials of the document or handwriting examiner used?
4. What is the status of the lawsuit, if any?
5. What evidence do you have that the notes have been forged?

These preliminary questions must be answered prior to opening a criminal investigation. As you know, time is of the essence due to possible statute of limitation issues.

I have written you instead of making a phone call for two reasons. One, I know you have talked with several people regarding this issue, and I don't want you to feel you have to "start from scratch" with me. The other reason is that I will need documentation regarding these questions, and a written request is easier to refer to than a telephone conversation. If you have any questions or concerns, please feel free to contact me either by phone or email.

Respectfully

Captain Joe Cawley

Detective Division

Idaho Falls Police Department

208 612-8654

V. M. Edwards [redacted]@gmail.com> Wed, Jun 5, 2013 at 8:18 AM
To: Joe Cawley [redacted]@idahofallsidaho.gov>
Cc: Mark McBride [redacted]@idahofallsidaho.gov>, Darren Cook [redacted]@idahofallsidaho.gov>

Good Morning,

I am sorry I could not respond on yesterday. I just took a position with a newspaper and was in training. I will send this information today, as I do realize time is of the essence. My original complaint was made on last year it was the police who refuse to look into it then. So I am aware of the the statue of limitations.

Sincerely,

Veverly Edwards
[Quoted text hidden]

V. M. Edwards [redacted]@gmail.com> Wed, Jun 5, 2013 at 9:06 AM
To: Joe Cawley [redacted]@idahofallsidaho.gov>
Cc: Mark McBride [redacted]@idahofallsidaho.gov>, Darren Cook [redacted]@idahofallsidaho.gov>

Mr. Cawley,

After reading your questions, it will more than likely take me more than a day to go through these files to identify when and where these documents were introduced during the proceedings. I am not trying to determined every time they were introduced but I do realize you need to determined if they were used. Also in these statutes (18-2601-2602) it is also a felony to use fraudulent information during the inquiry or investigative process of the trial/court proceeding, just wanted to point that out because I noticed that you only mentioned 'if they were introduced as evidence." I will get this done as expeditiously as possible, but i want to be accurate.

Again, thanks and I appreciate you investigating this issue.

Sincerely,

Veverly Edwards
[Quoted text hidden]

Joe Cawley <[redacted]@idahofallsidaho.gov> Wed, Jun 5, 2013 at 9:13 AM
To: "V. M. Edwards"[redacted]@gmail.com>

I realize this may take some time and I appreciate your desire to be accurate and complete. I will await your response, thank you.

From: V. M. Edwards [mailto:[redacted]@gmail.com]
Sent: Wednesday, June 05, 2013 10:07 AM
To: Joe Cawley
Cc: Mark McBride; Darren Cook
Subject: Re: Forgery Investigation

[Quoted text hidden]

V. M. Edwards <[redacted]@gmail.com> Mon, Jun 10, 2013 at 12:36 AM
To: Joe Cawley [redacted]@idahofallsidaho.gov>

Mr. Crawley,

My responses are below and I have attached documents to this email. I cannot attach the docs to one email. So I will send another with another set of documents

Responses to Forgery investigation:

1. Was the document(s) in question (the alleged forged notes) entered into evidence in a court proceeding?

   a. One of the documents was used during my deposition (I will send the page of the deposition and the doc). This was the document that G. Lance Nalder informed my ex-husband and I that weakened/compromised my testimony and one of the reasons he withdrew.

   b. The expert witness was given these documents to review to make his testimony to the court. He even identified the inconsistencies in Dr. Garland's reports.

   c. On July 25, 2012 I submitted to court and plaintiff a set of responses to requests for admissions and production of documents. Question 15 asked "Please produce any and all records, documents and evidence of any kind which supports your contention that any medical records in this case were altered, falsified or changed in any way? I presented the documents that Dr. Garland altered. I am attaching the documents that were filed in court.

2. If this document was submitted, when and who submitted it?

My deposition was done September of 2011.

Dr. [redacted] the expert witness testimony was filed with the court April 16, 2012 it was submitted by G. Lance Nalder

Veverly Edwards submitted response to question 15 above and documents requested to the court on July 25, 2012.

3. What is the name and credentials of the document or handwriting examiner used?

Jill Wilson-I am attaching her opinion and her resume is included

4. What is the status of the lawsuit, if any?

   Robyn's interests were dismissed without prejudice

5. What evidence do you have that the notes have been forged?

If a doctor writes a history of a medical condition into a patient's file there should be evidence that this happened in the past. Well, there is no evidence because Robyn never had migraine headaches. There is a registration document that I did fill out during Robyn's visit to Dr. Garland that asked for past medical history. I did not check anything on the list (a copy is included). Headaches/migraine was the first condition. I am an educated person and I know how to fill out a form. If I did not check it on my form, where would Dr. Garland come up with a history of this condition?

There is also a school form in the stack of court documents. Dr. Garland told me and Robyn that she had a rare form of migraine that caused numbness (Hemiplegic), not headaches. I told the school nurse what he told me and she wrote it on the document. She filled the top part of the document out the day of Robyn's appointment with Garland because I went back to the school to inform her of what he told us. I signed the next day because I had to get something in writing that stated he had instructed her on how to take the medication. There is also a note that is included that was attached to this form. You are not supposed to give Zomig for Hemiplegic migraines, which she did not have that condition either.

Robyn has been seen by a doctor at least once every year since birth, there is no history of migraine headaches in her medical file. Not one registration document in Dr. Garland's files with my handwriting on it suggests she even had a headache certainly not migraine headaches. He only saw her once. Her referral was for numbness in her limbs. Robyn had a numbing sensation while we were there not a headache. Robyn is competent and can speak for herself. Her short term memory was affected by the stroke.

Robyn had been seeing Dr. Moore at Idaho Falls Pediatrics for a several years. Dr. Moore or Porter has never seen her for a migraine headache. I am still going through the files to find her medical records prior to seeing Garland. I have them, just have a lot of boxes to go through. I could sign for you all to get copies from Idaho Falls Pediatrics.

She has other family members that lived with her (two brothers) if these headaches lasted all day, I would think it would be noticeable to others because it would have affected her ability to perform and attend activities and school. She has never been out of school for a headache. She was a very active student as well as other activities in the community. The school nurse at Eagle Rock Jr. High can testify to the fact that Robyn was not having migraine headaches because I spoke with her about Dr. Garland diagnosis her with a rare form of migraine that caused numbness instead of headaches. She should be able to testify to this because she knew Robyn. I have forgotten her name but I am sure the school district has records of who was assigned to Eagle Rock in October of 2007.

While I have attempted several times to get this address, I feel that someone in the police department has alliances or affiliations with this doctor and do not want him to be charged. I would never lie or attempt to destroy another person's character or reputation. Dr. Erich Garland falsified my child's medical records and then he and his attorney used them to make a mockery of Robyn's civil case against him.

Sincerely,

Veverly Edwards

On Tue, Jun 4, 2013 at 2:54 PM, Joe Cawley <[redacted]@idahofallsidaho.gov> wrote:
[Quoted text hidden]

---

2 attachments

court docs.pdf
9165K

expert witness testimony.pdf
6806K

V. M. Edwards <[redacted]@gmail.com> Mon, Jun 10, 2013 at 12:39 AM
To: Joe Cawley <[redacted]@idahofallsidaho.gov>

Here is the second set of docs.
[Quoted text hidden]

---

2 attachments

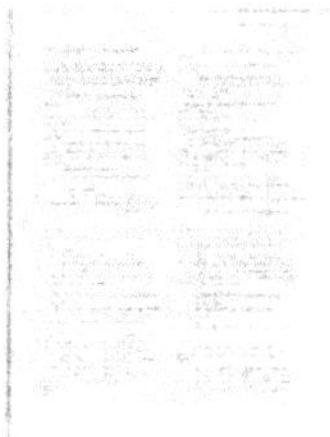

copy of deposition.jpg
566K

forensic expert opinion.pdf
9852K

1/19/2014 Gmail - (no subject)

Gmail

(no subject)

Joe Cawley @idahofallsidaho.gov> Mon, Jun 24, 2013 at 8:54 AM
To: "vevmyed@gmail.com" @gmail.com>

Ms. Edwards, there is not a case number as of yet. I still need the following information in order to determine if a criminal case is warranted. I noticed in your last reply you said "this is the second set of documents". I have a copy of the handwriting analysis and a copy of a deposition. If you sent any other documents, I have not received them. Thank you.

1. Was the document(s) in question (the alleged forged notes) entered into evidence in a court proceeding?
2. If this document was submitted, when and who submitted it?
4. What is the status of the lawsuit, if any?
5. What evidence do you have that the notes have been forged?

V. M. Edwards @gmail.com> Mon, Jun 24, 2013 at 9:14 AM
To: Joe Cawley @idahofallsidaho.gov>

I sent you several documents. Did you not receive them? And answered your questions.

Veverly
[Quoted text hidden]

V. M. Edwards @gmail.com> Mon, Jun 24, 2013 at 9:17 AM
To: Joe Cawley @idahofallsidaho.gov>

I responded to you on June 5th, should I forward the email to you that is in my sent folder.
[Quoted text hidden]

Joe Cawley @idahofallsidaho.gov> Mon, Jun 24, 2013 at 9:25 AM
To: "V. M. Edwards" @gmail.com>

I do have the correspondence from you dated June 5, there are no documents attached. The only correspondence I have with attachments are on June 10. If you tried to send additional items, I have not received them, so please do try again. Thanks.

Subject: Re:

[Quoted text hidden]

V. M. Edwards <@gmail.com> Mon, Jun 24, 2013 at 11:44 AM
To: Joe Cawley @idahofallsidaho.gov>

What did I send on June 10tb?

[Quoted text hidden]

V. M. Edwards @gmail.com> Mon, Jun 24, 2013 at 11:47 AM
To: Joe Cawley <@idahofallsidaho.gov>

I will resend the information, but I have it in my send folder where i sent attachments two separate emails because the attachments were large.
[Quoted text hidden]

Joe Cawley @idahofallsidaho.gov> Mon, Jun 24, 2013 at 12:20 PM
To: "V. M. Edwards" <@gmail.com>

On June 10 I received the questioned document examination and one page of a deposition. I'll wait for the rest and send you a confirmation when I receive them. Thanks.

From: V. M. Edwards [mailto@gmail.com]
Sent: Monday, June 24, 2013 12:47 PM
To: Joe Cawley
Subject: Re: Re:

[Quoted text hidden]

V. M. Edwards @gmail.com> Tue, Jun 25, 2013 at 8:56 AM
To: Joe Cawley @idahofallsidaho.gov>

Mr. Cawley,

Did you receive the email I sent on yesterday?

Veverly Edwards
[Quoted text hidden]

V. M. Edwards <@gmail.com> Tue, Jun 25, 2013 at 8:57 AM
To: Joe Cawley @idahofallsidaho.gov>

I sent it from my aol account.

Veverly Edwards
[Quoted text hidden]

Joe Cawley <@idahofallsidaho.gov> Tue, Jun 25, 2013 at 9:03 AM

To: "V. M. Edwards" [redacted]@gmail.com>

Sorry, no. I have not received anything from you containing any documents other than the handwriting analysis and a page from a deposition.

From: V. M. Edwards [mailto:[redacted]@gmail.com]
Sent: Tuesday, June 25, 2013 9:57 AM
To: Joe Cawley
Subject: Re: Re:

[Quoted text hidden]

V. M. Edwards <[redacted]@gmail.com> Tue, Jun 25, 2013 at 9:04 AM
To: Joe Cawley <[redacted]@idahofallsidaho.gov>

What is your fax number. I will fax it to you.

[Quoted text hidden]

Joe Cawley <[redacted]@idahofallsidaho.gov> Tue, Jun 25, 2013 at 9:05 AM
To: "V. M. Edwards" <[redacted]@gmail.com>

[redacted] Thank you.

From: V. M. Edwards [mailto:[redacted]@gmail.com]
Sent: Tuesday, June 25, 2013 10:05 AM
To: Joe Cawley
Subject: RE: Re:

[Quoted text hidden]

V. M. Edwards <[redacted]@gmail.com> Tue, Jun 25, 2013 at 10:09 AM
To: Joe Cawley <[redacted]@idahofallsidaho.gov>

My fax just confirmed 30 pages sent to 208-[redacted] Did you get them if not I will send them to someone I know there and have them to deliver them to you.

Veverly Edwards
[Quoted text hidden]

Joe Cawley <[redacted]@idahofallsidaho.gov> Tue, Jun 25, 2013 at 10:12 AM
To: "V. M. Edwards" <[redacted]@gmail.com>

Yes, they are coming through now. Let me examine the documents and present them to the prosecuting attorney for his review. I will be in touch with you as soon as possible.

From: V. M. Edwards [mailto:[redacted]@gmail.com]

Sent: Tuesday, June 25, 2013 11:09 AM

[Quoted text hidden]

[Quoted text hidden]

V. M. Edwards @gmail.com> Mon, Jul 22, 2013 at 6:48 AM
To: Joe Cawley @idahofallsidaho.gov>

Officer Cawley,

The last time we spoke I sent information to you and I was awaiting a response on a case number. I would like an update on where you are on my complaint against Dr. Garland falsifying information during a civil court proceeding?

Sincerely,

Veverly Edwards

On Mon, Jun 24, 2013 at 8:54 AM, Joe Cawley @idahofallsidaho.gov> wrote:
[Quoted text hidden]

Joe Cawley @idahofallsidaho.gov> Mon, Jul 22, 2013 at 7:18 AM
To: "V. M. Edwards" @gmail.com>

Ms. Edwards, this investigation was turned into the Bonneville Prosecuting Attorney on July 9, 2013. Once I receive a determination on how to proceed, I will contact you .

From: V. M. Edwards [mailto @gmail.com]
Sent: Monday, July 22, 2013 7:48 AM
To: Joe Cawley
Subject: Re:

Officer Cawley,

[Quoted text hidden]
[Quoted text hidden]

V. M. Edwards @gmail.com> Mon, Jul 22, 2013 at 7:26 AM
To: Joe Cawley @idahofallsidaho.gov>

So you do not have a case number for my complaint?
[Quoted text hidden]

Joe Cawley @idahofallsidaho.gov> Mon, Jul 22, 2013 at 7:30 AM
To: "V. M. Edwards" < @gmail.com>

Not yet. If the Prosecuting Attorney decides to proceed with criminal charges, a case number and court

1/19/2014 Gmail - (no subject)

number will be assigned at that time. If this is the case, I will email you as soon as I find out.

From: V. M. Edwards [mailto:[redacted]@gmail.com]
Sent: Monday, July 22, 2013 8:27 AM
To: Joe Cawley
Subject: Re: Re:

[Quoted text hidden]

V. M. Edwards <[redacted]@gmail.com> Mon, Jul 22, 2013 at 7:35 AM
To: Joe Cawley <[redacted]@idahofallsidaho.gov>

Officer Cawley

I don't mean to be worrisome, but I have had people to patronize me, attempt to intimidate me, and misinform myself and others. Is this norm as far as assigning case numbers? Just want to make sure I have my facts straight.

Veverly Edwards
[Quoted text hidden]

Joe Cawley <[redacted]@idahofallsidaho.gov> Mon, Jul 22, 2013 at 8:46 AM
To: "V. M. Edwards" <[redacted]@gmail.com>

I understand, no need to apologize. No, this is not the norm. Usually, in Detectives, we get cases from our patrol division and investigate specific crimes. In this instance, I was given this assignment after it had been through several different hands. I am not an attorney, so I do not know whether the documents you have provided offer enough evidentiary value for prosecution. If not, and I can further investigate the matter, then I will log a criminal case as with any other investigation. Right now, I'm looking for an expert legal determination as how to proceed.

From: V. M. Edwards [mailto:[redacted]@gmail.com]
Sent: Monday, July 22, 2013 8:35 AM

[Quoted text hidden]

[Quoted text hidden]

V. M. Edwards <[redacted]@gmail.com> Fri, Jul 26, 2013 at 3:02 PM
To: Joe Cawley <[redacted]@idahofallsidaho.gov>

Thanks for your response. So you have essentially done all you can and you are awaiting a response from the county prosecutor for direction, correct?

I am actually working on another news article and trying to get information on where my complaint is in the "justice process" and what the county prosecutor is doing because everyone seems to be dragging while the statute of limitations is running.

I have very little confidence in the justice system in Idaho Falls because it appears that integrity is lacking in many of the officials there.

https://mail.google.com/mail/u/0/?ui=2&ik=201ecf8ea7&view=pt&search=inbox&th=13f76e4672baff78 5/6

I do appreciate your responding.

Sincerely
Veverly Edwards
[Quoted text hidden]

1/19/2014 Gmail - Forgery Investigation

Gmail

Forgery Investigation

Joe Cawley [redacted]@idahofallsidaho.gov> Wed, Jul 31, 2013 at 11:12 AM
To: [redacted]@gmail.com" [redacted]@gmail.com>
Cc: Steve Barnes <[redacted]@idahofallsidaho.gov>

Ms. Edwards, the Prosecuting Attorney does not feel he has enough information for criminal prosecution at this time. I have assigned your case to Detective Steve Barnes. Detective Barnes has worked forgery and fraud cases for many years. He will be contacting you to obtain any further information he needs. He will also give you a case number. I will work with him and provide assistance as necessary.

V. M. Edwards [redacted]@gmail.com> Thu, Aug 1, 2013 at 7:28 AM
To: Joe Cawley <[redacted]@idahofallsidaho.gov>

Thanks Officer Cawley. I appreciate your assistance.

Veverly Edwards
[Quoted text hidden]

https://mail.google.com/mail/u/0/?ui=2&ik=201ecf8ea7&view=pt&search=inbox&th=14035ee7bc2b6c11 1/1

1/19/2014 Gmail - Fraud case

Gmail

Fraud case

Steve Barnes <[redacted]@idahofallsidaho.gov> Wed, Jul 31, 2013 at 10:44 A
To: "[redacted]@gmail.com" [redacted]@gmail.com>

Ms. Ververly Edwards,

I have been assigned the case you have requested and am in the process of doing an investigation. If you could call me I would appreciate it. I need to get some personal information from you to make the report.

I also have a couple of questions I would like to ask to assist my investigation. I am in and out of my office throughout the day, so if I am not in when you call, please leave me a message with your name and

Number, and I will call you back at my earliest convenience.

Sincerely,

Detective Steve Barnes

Idaho Falls Police

V. M. Edwards [redacted]@gmail.com> Thu, Aug 1, 2013 at 7:32 A
To: Steve Barnes <[redacted]@idahofallsidaho.gov>

Officer Barnes,

I am Veverly Edwards, Robyn Edwards mother, You may contact my cell phone [redacted]. Today, I will be in assessments with Robyn. I look forward to speaking with you.

Sincerely,

Veverly Edwards
[Quoted text hidden]

https://mail.google.com/mail/u/0/?ui=2&ik=201ecf8ea7&view=pt&search=inbox&th=14035d48f4ead10f

1/19/2014 Gmail - Investigation

Gmail

Investigation

V. M. Edwards [redacted]@gmail.com> Mon, Aug 19, 2013 at 10:59 AM
To: Steve Barnes [redacted]@idahofallsidaho.gov>

Officer Barnes,

I have a question, since you are investigating this. Dr. Garland references the MRI in that letter. If you requested the file from him, you would have the information regarding the dates and signatures in which he requested the MRI and it was scheduled, which would verify to you all, since the letter is being used as proof, that the letter was not written on October 1st. Did you even request her file from Dr. Garland?

I have a documented letter in which the prosecuting attorney and the city attorney agreed that it would not be "proper" mind you not legal but proper to prosecute Dr Garland for the felony he committed so I know that the prosecuting attorney is probably just going through the motions to see if I can come up with evidence, not that anyone is actually looking for the evidence but if I can come up with it to refute their efforts in trying not to prosecute because it is not "proper" and I wonder by what standard they are measuring who it is proper to prosecute for a felony offense?

I have no doubt that they all know that Dr. Garland is guilty but for whatever discriminating factors, have decided to pretend that the evidence is not there, when I know it is because I have seen the documents. I will work on getting emails and copies of the documents that you should have received from Dr. Garland that is if you all have requested any from him.

Again I don't mean to sound harsh, but I know what I am up against and it has nothing to do with right or wrong or justice.

Sincerely,

Veverly Edwards

Steve Barnes [redacted]@idahofallsidaho.gov> Mon, Aug 19, 2013 at 11:44 AM
To: "V. M. Edwards" [redacted]@gmail.com>

I understand what you are saying, and doing all I can. I am not trying to push you away. If you are able to come up with anything further to help, I will do what I can.

Thank You!

Detective Steve Barnes

From: V. M. Edwards [mailto:[redacted]@gmail.com]
Sent: Monday, August 19, 2013 11:59 AM

https://mail.google.com/mail/u/0/?ui=2&ik=201ecf8ea7&view=pt&search=inbox&th=14097baf11ef7799 1/2

1/19/2014 Gmail - Investigation

To: Steve Barnes
Subject: Investigation

[Quoted text hidden]

V. M. Edwards <[redacted]@gmail.com> Mon, Aug 19, 2013 at 11:59 AM
To: Steve Barnes <[redacted]@idahofallsidaho.gov>

Officer Barnes,

I appreciate what you have done, but I have dealt with your superiors and I know that the concept of justice for "all" escapes them.

[Quoted text hidden]

V. M. Edwards [redacted]@gmail.com> Mon, Aug 19, 2013 at 6:00 PM
To: Steve Barnes <[redacted]@idahofallsidaho.gov>
Cc: [redacted], [redacted]n

Officer Barnes,

While I was searching through my files,I thought about two witnesses that I spoke with the evening of October 1st, 2007. I spoke with Robyn's father,[redacted], who is a registered nurse and my sister, [redacted] who is also a registered nurse and they both questioned why an MRI was not ordered.

I copied them on this letter because they encouraged me to get one ordered. You can get information from either of them because I was in contact with them both.

I am sure both of them would be willing to talk to you.

Sincerely,

Veverly Edwards
[Quoted text hidden]

https://mail.google.com/mail/u/0/?ui=2&ik=201ecf8ea7&view=pt&search=inbox&th=14097baf11ef7799 2/

Gmail

Fraud Investigation

V. M. Edwards [redacted]@gmail.com> Thu, Sep 12, 2013 at 8:29 AM
To: Steve Barnes [redacted]@idahofallsidaho.gov>

Officer Barnes,

Did you received the medical records I emailed to you? You did not respond. I also sent you information on two witnesses.

I am not sure how the Idaho Falls Police handle investigations into fraud, but I fail to see how it can be done without a careful examination of the records and those connected to the events that transpired.

I will await your response.

Sincerely,

Veverly Edwards

Steve Barnes [redacted]@idahofallsidaho.gov> Thu, Sep 12, 2013 at 8:34 AM
To: "V. M. Edwards" [redacted]@gmail.com>

Yes I received the information.

From: V. M. Edwards [mailto[redacted]@gmail.com]
Sent: Thursday, September 12, 2013 9:29 AM
To: Steve Barnes
Subject: Fraud Investigation

[Quoted text hidden]

V. M. Edwards [redacted]@gmail.com> Sat, Nov 30, 2013 at 2:28 PM
To: Steve Barnes [redacted]@idahofallsidaho.gov>

Officer Barnes,

I have not heard from you since I sent the names of two witnesses who can verify the information contained in the letter written on October 1, 2007 was fraudulent. The MRI was ordered on the second. After speaking with my ex-husband and my sister regarding the appointment earlier in the day on Ocober 1, 2007 they agreed that an MRI was needed. I requested the MRI on October 2, 2007. So how would Garland have information about it in a letter he states he wrote on October 1, 2007. The letter is another piece to show his fraudulent activities. Did you call these individuals for statements? You said you needed additional information, they can verify my statement.

Please let me know the status of the investigation.

Sincerely,

https://mail.google.com/mail/u/0/?ui=2&ik=201ecf6ea7&view=pt&search=inbox&th=14112ca28b10159b 1/2

Veverly Edwards
[Quoted text hidden]

V. M. Edwards[redacted]@gmail.com> Tue, Dec 3, 2013 at 4:30 PM
To: Joe Cawley <[redacted]@idahofallsidaho.gov>

Officer Cawley,

I have attempted to contact Officer Barnes but he is not responding. I have not heard from him since I sent him information on two witnesses. He did not contact them, so I am wondering where the status of the case.

Sincerely,

Veverly Edwards
[Quoted text hidden]

1/19/2014 Gmail - Fraud Investigation/Additional Information

Gmail

Fraud Investigation/Additional Information

V. M. Edwards <[redacted]@gmail.com> Sun, Dec 29, 2013 at 9:55 PM
To: Steve Barnes [redacted]@idahofallsidaho.gov>, Joe Cawley [redacted]@idahofallsidaho.gov>

While you all appear to have discontinued the investigation into my complaint and refused to reply to my inquiries, I have not stopped investigating it. I am attaching the copies of the complaints I filed on last year against G. Lance Nalder, Breck Barton and Dr. Erich Garland.

I am also attaching a letter from Mr. Nalder regarding his reasoning for withdrawing from the case. He actually lied on me and the expert witness. I am also forwarding a statement from the expert witness denying he ever changed his testimony. Mr. Nalder stated to my ex-husband and I that the expert recanted his testimony. Mr. Nalder has also lied to others to keep this case from going forward. He has portrayed me as someone who is distraught and misguided.

I informed you all last year of their attempts to undermined my daughter's case. If the malpractice case had no merit, why would Mr. Nalder and Mr. Barton attempt to intimidate me with fraudulent medical records from Dr. Garland and lie on the expert witness?

Officer Barnes, you asked if I had any additional information. Well, I am sending it to you. These individuals have made a mockery of the civil court process and committed felony offenses in which you all refuse to investigate.

I imagine you all think you are frustrating me, but you are not. I am more determined to seek justice and I am sure that when it is all over, many people will be exposed for their part in this gross miscarriage of justice.

Sincerely,

Veverly Edwards

2 attachments

Letter from Nalder regarding withdrawing0001.pdf
1646K

[redacted]Ltr 11-11-13.pdf
203K

https://mail.google.com/mail/u/0/?ui=2&ik=201ecf8ea7&view=pt&search=sent&th=14342128832f1038 1/1

Epilogue

The Lord God is my strength, and he will make my feet like hinds' feet, and he will make me to walk upon mine high places...

Habakkuk 3:19 (KJV)

While I would like to think situations like Robyn's are rare, they are not. Thousands of patients die each year due to preventable medical errors and millions are affected. Many, like Robyn, are left disabled for life. It is time for the governing bodies of this nation to do more to protect patients and families against doctors like Dr. Erich Garland, and the corrupt communities that protect them. Their actions were inhumane. What kind of doctor changes a child's medical records in an attempt to undermine the child and her mother? What kind of lawyer undermines his client's case? What does this say about the legal and medical communities in Idaho that protect such individuals? What are the consequences for the citizens in states like Idaho?

The basic inalienable rights of life, liberty and the pursuit of happiness were stripped from Robyn, and the culprit has been cuddled and protected by the criminal minds of the justice system in Idaho. I believe President Obama made a very profound statement in his inaugural address January 21, 2013:

> "Today we continue a never-ending journey to bridge the meaning of those words with the realities of our time. For history tells us that while these truths may be self-evident, they've never been self-executing; that while freedom is a gift from God, it must be secured by His people here on Earth. The patriots of 1776 did not fight to replace the tyranny of a king with the privileges of a few or the rule of a mob. They gave to us a republic, a government of, and by, and for the people, entrusting each generation to keep safe our founding creed."

It appears that justice will prevail in Robyn's case, only if an investigation is launched by the federal government into the actions of the officials in Idaho Falls and Boise, Idaho, who took part in this gross miscarriage of justice. I imagine that Robyn was not the first minority patient in Idaho to be stripped of her basic human rights of life, liberty and the pursuit of happiness, and her right to civil recourse. I assume that the reason these individuals attempted this cruel act is because they have been successful in the past.

In addition to that, Idaho Statue 6 – 1012, Proof of Community Standard of Heath in Malpractice Cases, should be stricken from use. This standard is a breeding ground for corrupt practices. Dr. Erich Garland was the initiator of the fraudulent acts in Robyn's case. He was the first to add false information to her medical records. Then a doctor from here primary care physician's office followed his lead by adding false information to the records at that location. I presume this was done to establish a medical history of migraine headaches. It appears that making false entries into patient's medical records after negligence has occurred is common practice in Idaho Falls. I guess this would be considered "Proof of Community Standard of Health Care" in Idaho. This statute essentially allows doctors to create their own standard of medical care, and violate the rights of the patients and their families. Consequently patients and families are written off as being misguided.

Given Robyn's situation and others who have fallen prey to these practices, I would ask that the section of the Patient Protection and Affordable Care Act pertaining to Medical Malpractice be re-evaluated. I suggest a national health care standard. If this does not change at the national level, minority patients and may others will continue to be victims to negligent doctors because there is no on to protect them against medical communities like the one that exists in Idaho Falls, Idaho.

Robyn was a child just starting to realize her abilities, and excited about life. She had high hopes and dreams. She was an honor student with a lot of potential. I realize in order for the officials in Idaho to apply the law justly, they must first recognize Robyn as a human being like themselves. This is difficult, almost impossible to do, when those administering the law have lived their lives eating and digesting distorted information about African Americans and other minorities, and with an even greater distortion of their own self-worth.

I recently sat and watched "A Time to Kill." Even though I watched this movie many times in the past, this time the meaning truly hit home. As I watched and examined the theme, I was totally enthralled by the movie. Near the end of the movie, the white attorney representing the black defendant is asked to examine his own prejudices. After examining himself, in his closing remarks he presented the same request to the jurors. He asked the jurors to close their eyes and imagine the little black girl who had been beaten and raped, was actually a little white girl. Unlike this fictional movie, we did not find a lawyer in courageous enough to take on the criminals within the Idaho judicial system.

Every time I read about another family in the news fighting a battle similar to ours, I realize that this book needs to be published. Many families are facing the same discriminatory practices, where medical officials change medical records and attempt to make the family look misguided. The patients and families who stand against these practices are written off. There is no defense for patients against organizations that are vulnerable to the unlawful practices of those who regulate their systems.

In Robyn's case, the officials in Idaho are waiting us out. They know the statute of limitations is running out on Robyn's case, and their fraudulent acts. So they have continued to ignore my request for a formal investigation. The police made it appear that they were investigating. But as the evidence shows in this book, had they actually conducted an investigation they would have uncovered the same information that I discovered. Unless the federal government steps in, the violations of Robyn's basic human rights will not be addressed.

Robyn Oneida Edwards is my only daughter. The evil spirits of men, who have no respect for humanity, destroyed her life. God saw it all, and I have to believe that in His infinite wisdom, He left her here to be a voice for many who have come against the same evil in the civil and criminal justice system in Idaho. It is imperative that the governing bodies of this nation address the lack of ethics in the medical and legal arena as it relates to medical malpractice. The lives of patients are at stake. A mob, the good ole boy network, should not possess the power to disarm the laws and statutes at their discretion to cover for one of their negligent doctors.

Robyn graduated high school in May of 2012. She now attends a program for people with Acquired Brain Injuries. She graduates from the brain injury program in May of 2014, and plans to attend college in the fall of 2014. The plan is to take one class a semester. We are not in a hurry. We will trust God as we continue on this journey, step by step, one day at a time.

For I know the plans I have for you, declares the Lord,plans to prosper you and not to harm you, and plans to give you hope and a future.

Jeremiah 29:11 (NIV)

—— ✧ ——

A Mother and Daughter's Appeal to National Officials and U.S. Citizens

President Obama, I appeal to you, the Senate and the Congress of the United States to reform the medical malpractice torts and to create a national standard of medical care. I recently downloaded a copy of the Patient Protection and Affordable Care Act. I applaud you for providing affordable care to all Americans. However, I was disappointed when I read the Sense of the Senate on Medical Malpractice reform. It seemed to me the states are basically given an option as to whetherthey reform their medical malpractice statutes. This book is a testament to what happens when a mop of corrupt men have the liberty to create and administer laws at their will. You must know that places like Idaho will not willingly protect the rights of "all" patients and families.

I recently read Idaho's Senate Bill 1355 (Sixty Second Legislature/Second Regular Session of 2014) created in reference to the Patient Protection and Affordable Care Act (PPACA). Their sixty second legislature referenced, "P.L. 111-148 of the PPACA."

It basically establishes that Idaho does not adhere to any standards of medical care outside of their own, which is a scary thought considering what happened to Robyn. There are doctors and facilities in Idaho that operate at a substandard level, yet, they are allowed to use high potency drugs and equipment which can destroy and debilitate patients. This is what concerns and dismays me. President Obama, it is not fair to patients and families to allow states to create medical communities that operate at a substandard level of medical care. This violates the patient's basic human rights of life, liberty and the pursuit of happiness.

President Obama, I hope that you, the Senate and Congress will re-evaluate the sections of the PPACA on medical Malpractice and develop a national standard of medical care, and definitive laws that govern the states on medical malpractice, because if you do not I am afraid to consider the outcome for many patients and their families.

U.S. Attorney General Eric Holder, I also appeal to you. What these Idaho officials did under the auspices of justice was clearly a violation of my daughter's basic human rights. To make it even worse, their licensing boards also took part in the conspiracy. I pray that you authorize a federal investigation into the actions of the judge presiding over Robyn's case, the lawyers, the Idaho Bar Association, the FBI Boise location, the Idaho Attorney General's Office, the Bonneville County Prosecutor and the Idaho Falls Police Department. It these inhumane acts are not addressed, innocent lives will continue to be destroyed, and wrong will continue to appear right in the eyes of the oppressor in Idaho.

Secretary of the Department of Health and Human Services, I appeal to you too. In the past, there have been complaints against the Idaho Board of Medicine for failure to discipline negligent doctors. Surely, there is some action that can be taken by your department to ensure that medical boards, like the one in Idaho, do not continue to allow these negligent doctors to practice while covering for their atrocious violations.

Accountability in medical care cannot be an option. Discrimination is alive and well in the United States and it operates behind a smoke screen. The only reason I was able to acquire the information that I placed in this book is because I took on the legal case myself. The attorneys representing Robyn's case were not threatened by giving me this information. They knew that every road I took for recourse in Idaho was already tainted with unjust men, their partners in crime. Most patients are not able to obtain the information that I collected. I believe it was God's will that I did, and that I share Robyn's story to ensure other patients do not fall victim to medical communities like those that exist in Idaho.

I compel every citizen in this nation to find out what the statutes are in their states pertaining to patient care and medical malpractice. Like many of you, before Robyn's ordeal, I worked, paid my insurance premiums, and was content. I could have never imagined all that transpired in Idaho from 2007 - 2012.

Patients and families, you need to find out where your elected officials stand on this subject, especially those in Idaho. Use your votes to voice your concerns. We cannot afford to elect officials who continuously promote statutes that are substandard and that clearly violate the basic human rights of citizens in the U.S.

While I make these appeals, I am aware that some men are only subject to their own selfish ambitions. I am not moved by rejection. My faith is rooted in the Lord.

> [35] *Who shall separate us from the love of Christ? Shall trouble or hardship*

or persecution or famine or nakedness or danger or sword? [36] As it is written:

"For your sake we face death all day long: we are considered as sheep to be slaughtered" [37] No, in all these things we are more than conquerors through him who loved us. [38] For I am convinced that neither death nor life, neither angels nor demons, neither present nor the future, nor any powers, [39] neither height nor depth, nor anything else in all creation, will be able to separate us from the love of God that is in Christ Jesus our Lord. Romans 8: 35-39 (NIV)

Notes

Chapter – 3 Dr. Erich Garland and the Idaho Board of Medicine

1. Dafer, Rima M. “Migraine Variants.” 29 March 2012. Medscape. <http://emedicine.medscape.com/article/1142731-overview>

2. Garcia, Richard S. “The Misuse of Race in Medical Diagnosis.” *Pediatrics* 113 (2004): 1394-1395. PDF file.

3. Garland, Erich Dep. pg. 25:8, 14-16, 23-25, pg. 71: 11-14.

4. Holland, Kimberly. “Rare and Extreme Types of Migraine's.” 1 July 2013. Healthline. < http://www.healthline.com/health/migraine-rare-and-extreme-types-of-migraines>

5. Public Citizen Protecting Health, Safety and Democracy. “New Public Citizen Study Questions Ability of State Medical Boards to Protect Patients From Dangerous Doctors." **15 March 2011.** http://www.citizen.org/pressroom/pressroomredirect.cfm?ID=3294

6. WebMD. “What is a Migraine with Aura?” Migraines and Headaches Health Center. 25 February 2013. http://www.webmd.com/migraines-headaches/what-is-a-migraine-with-aura

7. Zomig tablets and Zomig-ZMT Orally Disintegrating Tablets. US Food and Drug Administration. September 2012. <http://www.accessdata.fda.gov/drugsatfda_docs/label/2012/020768s019s021,021231s010s011lbl.pdf>

Chapter – 4 G. Lance Nalder and the Idaho Bar Association

1. Idaho Rules of Professional Conduct. Preamble: A Lawyers Responsibilities. Idaho State Bar. 1 July 2004. PDf file. <http://isb.idaho.gov/pdf/rules/irpc.pdf>

Chapter – 6 Corruption Among Idaho Falls Officials

1. Desirai Schild. "Get to know F.A.S.T. It may save your life." Post Register's Eastern Idaho Medical Guide. Spring-Summer 2012. Idaho Falls, Idaho.

2. Falsifying Evidence. Evidence Falsified or Concealed and Witnesses Intimidated or Bribed. State of Idaho Legislature, Idaho Statutes, Title 18 Crimes and Punishments. 18-2601, 1972. http://legislature.idaho.gov/idstat/Title18/T18CH26SECT18-2601.htm

3. Preparing False Evidence. Evidence Falsified or Concealed and Witnesses Intimidated or Bribed. State of Idaho Legislature, Idaho Statutes, Title 18 Crimes and Punishments. 18-2602, 1972. http://legislature.idaho.gov/idstat/Title18/T18CH26SECT18-2602.htm

Chapter – 7 Epilogue

1. Obama, Barack. "Inaugural Address 2013," President's Inauguration, Washington D.C. 21 Jan. 2013. http://www.whitehouse.gov/the-press-office/2013/01/21/inaugural-address-president-barack-obama

Appendix

The following pages are an eight-page testimony from the expert witness who Attorney Lance Nalder's law firm retained for Robyn Edwards' medical malpractice case. Attorney Nalder gave testimony to the Idaho Bar Association that Dr. Lombardi withdrew his testimony, but Dr. Lombardi did not withdraw his testimony. It appears that the Idaho Bar Association never contacted Dr. Lombardi to verify the statement even though they used it as a reason not to hold him responsible for defrauding Robyn Edwards' medical malpractice case.

As a Black mother, even with a substantial amount of evidence, without honest people to provide oversight on professional regulatory boards, police departments, and judicial processes, voices like mine are silenced by systemic racism.

David A. Lombardi, M.D.

DIPLOMATE AMERICAN BOARD OF NEUROLOGY

MEDICAL NEUROLOGY
ELECTROENCEPHALOGRAPHY
ELECTROMYOGRAPHY

1467 NORTH WANDA ROAD, SUITE 165
ORANGE, CALIFORNIA 92867
TELEPHONE (714) 289-1240
FAX (714) 289-1276

March 22, 2012

Benjamin Mason, Esq.
Nalder Law Office
591 Park Avenue, Suite 201
Idaho Falls, ID 83402

RE: EDWARDS, ROBYN

This dictation is to memorialize our phone conversation of March 21, 2012, regarding my review of additional medical records and opinion on Robyn Edwards. I previously had dictated an opinion about previous review of records on January 11, 2010, concerning this 13-year-old female. At that time, my review of records indicated that this 13-year-old female presented to Erich W. Garland, M.D., a neurologist, on October 1, 2007, with symptoms of migraine-like headaches and episodes of hemiparesis specifically involving the left face, arm, and leg. The patient had an episode prior to being evaluated by this neurologist in his office just prior to the office visit. In that dictation, I indicated that the doctor indicates, "She will get numbness in the left face, arm and leg, and sometimes have weakness in the left arm and leg lasting as long as an hour." The exam by the time she reached his office was normal. Dr. Garland made the diagnosis of migraine headaches and prescribed oral triptan. An MRI of the brain was ordered. Unfortunately, she used the triptan and before the MRI was performed, she developed a right hemispheric infarction. She was subsequently found to have Moyamoya. The onset of her stroke was approximately 12:45 p.m. on October 4, 2007. She was admitted at that time and had workup including CT and MRI scans that diagnosed an abnormality and she was transferred to Primary Children's Medical Center in Salt Lake City. Since that dictation, I have received additional medical records for my review. I also re-reviewed the medical records received by me on a CD entitled Robyn Edwards Medical Summary as well as the transcript of the testimony of a deposition on Erich W. Garland. That deposition was on January 14, 2011. It was 78 pages long and it was reviewed in its entirety. The additional medical records are the deposition of Robert Edwards, the patient's father, dated September 22, 2011, which is 70 pages long and was reviewed in its entirety. Additionally, there is a deposition of Veverly Edwards, the patient's mother, which was 200 pages long and was reviewed in its entirety.

After reviewing the above medical records, including the new medical records, I would like to make the following comments. In the deposition of Robert Edwards (the patient's father), on page 19 and page 20, in reference to a question concerning any communications with Veverly about Robyn and her health before she had the stroke, he indicated, "I recall her having a

RE: EDWARDS, ROBYN
March 22, 2012
Page 2

doctor's appointment and getting referred to a neurologist because she was having some numbness" that was intermittent, that they could not really relate to any triggers but the fact that there was numbness was a real concern for me. Q: Why is that? A: I am thinking TIA, a transient ischemic attack. On page 22 and 23 of that deposition, when he was asked if he had had any conversation with Robyn about this numbness issue, he related that in a phone conversation she said she did not feel like going to school that day. He believed this conversation was after she had seen the neurologist. Q: When she said she did not feel like she was going to school, what did she tell you? A: It was very difficult to pin her down. What I was getting from it was that there was some numbness issue and then she would feel weak too. Q: Do you remember her saying she was numb? A: She used the word "numb and tingly." He states that in a discussion with Veverly about Robyn about the visit with Dr. Garland, she indicated, "He did an examination and said that she had some type of migraine condition. He wanted to start her on medications. I asked her if there was any blood work drawn or anything down prior to arriving at the conclusion to start with medication, especially the types of medication. Q: Did you suggest he do anything else? A: We discussed an MRI as a baseline. This child was having symptoms. We don't know what they are. Before we give medication to mask those symptoms, we need to have a baseline of what's going on with her. That was the issue. He denied any health issues himself with migraine and no migraine in his family. Throughout that entire deposition, there is no mention of headaches accompanying the numbness episodes.

In Veverly Edwards deposition, on page 63, Q: So Robyn came home about the middle of August of 2007, correct? A: From the summer visit, yes (with her father). Q: And you are saying sometime between when she came home and before her stroke, she had complaints of numbness that you called and talked to her about? A: Yes. She had some numbness in her leg. She was not certain which leg. In early part of the year, she told me her elbow once felt some numbness (page 66). This was January or February 2007. On page 69 and 70, an episode is described in which she was at the rec center playing ball and was out on the floor playing ball and her right side went numb. She was playing basketball. It was just her right hand that went numb. Page 73, summarized, so again, she had just those three episodes that you are aware of and any memory off. She had numbness, one was elbow, one was leg, one was right hand. They indicate the patient is right hand dominant. This is page 82. They talk about her residuals from her stroke with cognitive losses of memory. Her cognitive skills were affected. She can was with a brace but she cannot run. She is not able to do much of anything with her left arm. She has left neglect on the left side in her peripheral vision. She has a manual wheelchair but someone has to push it. She cannot see to the left side. On page 114, Q: If I understand correctly from your memory of what you have said to me, this numbness issue wasn't something that happened on a daily basis, it had only happened a few isolated times before? A: Yes. Q: Did Robyn take medication of any kind for any reason before this happened in October 2007? A: No, multivitamins was all. Q: So no aspirin, no Tylenol. A: No. I can't think of anything she would have taken it for. On page 118, Q: So you show up at Dr. Garland. Tell me what you remember that day. A: It was raining that day. We pulled up in the parking lot. Just as we

18

RE: EDWARDS, ROBYN
March 22, 2012
Page 4

any complaints? A: Yes. She was experiencing numbness in one of her legs. I gave her a Zomig. She is not certain which leg. Q: What happens next? A: She was feeling better. So I left her and went back to work. She states she left work at noon, came home for lunch and went back to work. I decided to take the rest of the afternoon off of work and went back home. Robyn and I were going to go out, for I told her, let's go out. I needed to find some more mattresses. I asked how she was feeling. She said, I'm fine. We left then and I went to pick up a friend. My friend asked me to take her keys into her daughter. Robyn took them in and I noticed her getting kind of -- her gait was wobbly. I asked her if she was okay and she said yeah, saying she is feeling fine. She estimates that she left work around 1:30 or so and got home around 2:00. Page 157, Q: Okay, so you and your daughter go to look at mattresses. You stop to pick up one of your friends, Loretta Westbrook. And Robyn, when she got out of the car, you observed something was off with her gait. A: Yes, she was wobbly. I looked at her and said, you need to get back to the car. She said, but I need to take the keys in. I said, no, you need to get into the car. She got into the car. I think we will just go home. At that time, she said, I got a headache. Dr. Garland told me if she gets a headache, I give her ibuprofen. She lied down on the couch at home. She got up a couple of hours later, maybe 5:00 or 6:00 o'clock and she said, mom, I'm weak on my left side, can you help me to the bed. She got into the bed and went back to sleep. No, first she asked to lie down with her. I lied down in bed with her. I guess we got up at 10:00 or 11:00 o'clock. She said, mom, I can't move my left side. I got her up, I helped her get dressed. I asked my son to take her to the car and we went to the emergency room. (**My comment**: The emergency room check in sheet says the time they arrived was 0041 hours.) Page 163, Again Veverly denies that her daughter had headaches associated with her numbness symptoms. She indicates on page 167 that, I don't know that I gave her another Zomig that evening (October 4th) when she told me she was still weak, I don't know. Page 168, Q: So the record is clear, she took one around noon of the Zomig, just one pill. A: Yes. Q: Then she took the ibuprofen around 4:00. A: Yes. Q: And you don't know whether she took another Zomig before going to the hospital or not? A: No, I don't recall. Q: (By Mr. Jones), You are saying that Robyn reported to you later on that she had taken these three Zomig. When did she report this to you? A: Later, after I asked her -- she said she had taken three. I don't know when she took them. I don't know. I can't tell you. I don't know. Obviously I did not know she had taken those others. Page 170, Q: So if we back up then, how many of these Zomig pills she took? One was on the first at Dr. Garland's office. A: Yes. Q: One was the evening of the first. A: Yes. Q: One was at noon on the fourth. A: Yes. Q: There may have been one in the evening of the fourth, and you are understanding that there are three others at sometime. A: Yeah, I don't know what she was counting. (**My comment**: Therefore, between October 1st and the patient's stroke, she took three or four that are accounted for and possibly another three, so a total of possibly six or seven Zomig between 10/01/2007 and 10/04/2007.) In the rest of the deposition, they talk about them being airlifted out to Salt Lake City. They told me she had Moyamoya. The right side was completely stroke so there was no reason to do the bypass that they did on the left side. They wouldn't be able to do the left side until she got the swelling down. Q: So going forward, once you arrived in Salt Lake, your daughter was evaluated and your understanding was to (a) get the swelling down to and if we make through that okay, then (b) address some effort to

RE: EDWARDS, ROBYN
March 22, 2012
Page 5

include vascularization of the left side of the brain. A: Yes. Robyn probably woke up at the very end of October going into November. She opened her eyes about the 17th, but there was nothing there. So roughly 30 days into this, she started to see signs of improvement. They took her home at the end of January or February 2008. At that time she could not walk, could not feed herself. She would need a total care. In August or September, I changed her physical therapy to water therapy. In January 2009, we took her back to Primary to get extensive physical therapy, and she stayed there a month.

In Dr. Garland's deposition, there are discrepancies between what he says in his deposition and what is documented in the hospital records from Eastern Idaho Regional Medical Center. On page 25, he states, well, the mother reported that she had headaches for two to three months. They were, she recovered completely between the spells. She would have multiple spells that were brief five to ten minutes or less. Headaches would usually occur as the spell resolved. She had no visual changes. She had fatigue and numbness of her upper and lower <u>extremities</u>. In his dictation of October 5, 2007, at Eastern Idaho Regional Medical Center, his history is that the patient is a 13-year-old African-American right-handed female who was first seen by me on October 1, 2007, with recurrent episodes of headache, much worse in the past two months, which usually with the sense of disequilibrium and sometimes vertigo. Headaches occur after a spell. Most spells are brief, usually five to ten minutes, not associated with visual change. She would get fatigue, which can last hours or for the rest of the day. Spells can occur more than once a day. Nausea occurs occasionally but there is no vomiting. She had a brief episode prior to her exam in my office on October 1, 2007. She would get numbness in her face, arm and leg, and sometimes will have weakness in the left arm, leg, lasting as long as an hour. (**<u>My comment</u>**: The deposition indicates headaches with numbness of the upper and lower extremities, but his dictation of 10/05/2007 says the symptoms are lateralized to the left with left sided face, arm and leg numbness and weakness.) On page 27, they ask him, what are the classic symptoms of a migraine? He indicates, well, migraines can vary but you get symptoms that are reoccurring and you recover between the spells. Headache is present most of the time. You can have mood changes, fatigue, numbness. Sometimes you have visual distortion. You can have problems with expression and word finding, fatigue, generalized weakness is sometimes common. You only have a few of the symptoms though to call it a migraine. (**<u>My comment</u>**: Numbness, word finding difficulty, problems with expression are definitely not compatible with a classical migraine.) On page 29, line 13, Q: And you said numbness in the extremities is a classical migraine symptom? A: Yes. (**<u>My comment</u>**: It is not.) On page 34 and 35, Q: Do you remember some of those contraindications listed for Zomig? A: We don't use it in people with heart disease or people who have had a stroke or people with high blood pressure. Q: Do you know why you don't use in people who had strokes? A: My understanding is when the triptans came out, the FDA put the same restrictions they did for ergots and ergots were thought to be peripheral vasoconstrictive so they put that labeling on all the triptan drugs although there is no evidence they have ever caused a stroke. Page 37, Q: Does the FDA still require that for Zomig? A: They have not-- they have never changed the warning or contraindication labels because there have never been any studies to prove either way. On page 39, they refer to a letter that

RE: EDWARDS, ROBYN
March 22, 2012
Page 6

Dr. Garland had written to Dr. Porter indicating that because of some unusual features of her headaches, will get an MRI of the brain. She had numbness in both arms and legs, and she did not have any visual distortion. Other than that, it was pretty common for all of her symptoms to be migraine. Q: So what was unusual about that? A: The numbness usually occurs only on one side of the body. He said that what was unusual, was the numbness was on both sides of the body, which is the way presented in her, and then the absence of visual symptoms was unusual for migraine. Although you don't have to have either one. Q: But the presence of numbness does not rule out a migraine? A: The presence of numbness is common for migraine. If she did not have numbness, you can still have migraine, but usually they have some other symptoms. (<u>**My comment**</u>: I disagree with this series of answers.) On page 41 of the deposition, they review the prescription for the MRI. He states he instructed the staff to send it to Teton Radiology. Q: There under the principal diagnosis/symptoms it says, "atypical migraine." A: Right. He says, I think what I probably put in, what I coded it, which was migraine -- I put migraine variant, which is atypical migraine. That's because she had numbness on both sides of her body and extreme fatigue and a lack of visual symptoms, that's why I called it atypical migraine. Q: Did you consider doing an MRI on the 1st, when you were meeting with Robyn? A: Yes, I considered but told the patient and her mother that because her exam was normal, she had had symptoms for three months, and I did not think brain imaging was indicated at that time. (<u>**My comment**</u>: This totally ignores the patient's history.) On page 43, I said I did not think the MRI was needed because there was no clinical indication for it at the time of the first visit, and that if they wanted to do it -- sometimes just having the knowledge that you have a normal MRI is reassuring the management of the patient. (<u>**My comment**</u>: Atypical migraine is a clinical indication for doing an MRI.) On page 45, Q: Are you familiar with a test called an MRA? A: Yes. Q: How is that different from the MRI? A: It requires contract and they use the speed of blood flow to perform images. (<u>**My comment**</u>: MRAs of the brain do not require contrast enhancement, only MRAs of the neck do.) He goes on to state that MR angiograms are not required in someone with suspected migraine or even headaches. An MRA would be done looking for aneurysms or vessel blockages, and that's going to be someone you think is having a stroke. (<u>**My comment**</u>: How about vascular malformations or transient ischemic attacks.) He goes on to states that when she was in the hospital, the MRI showed acute right MCA stroke. On page 69, they ask him if he is familiar with the term "transient ischemic attack." His answer is yes. That means transient episodes of loss of brain function that can be migraine, strokes, seizures, cardiac events, hypoglycemia and there is a big differential for TIA. His answer is that is a subset of a stroke. On page 73 and 74, Q: Okay, do you know of any precautions that would have prevented her stroke? A: Well, she was young. I mean, stroke is extremely unusual in young people. She did not have any symptoms that were suggestive of a stroke or making a stroke high end differential. It was low. So you know, she was treated on the premise she had a migraine. (<u>**My comment**</u>: In his dictation of 10/05/2007, he indicates that she had episodes of numbness of her left face, arm and leg, and sometimes weakness of the left arm and leg lasting as long as an hour. This is a description certainly compatible with a transient ischemic attack, which Dr. Garland in his deposition says is a subset of a stroke.) On page 74, Q: Just so I'm clear, we talked about her symptoms of numbness in the extremities and weakness. Is it your

RE: EDWARDS, ROBYN
March 22, 2012
Page 7

recollection that the weakness and numbness was on both sides until her presentation at EIRMC on the night of the 4th? A: She had numbness on both sides. When she was in the office, on the 1st, she did not talk, did not complain of weakness or talked of it. You know, she talked more of fatigue. She said it was on both sides. The weakness wasn't diagnosed until she was in the hospital on the 5th. (**My comment**: Again, see his dictation of 10/05/2007.) Page 77, Q: We just discussed the symptoms that were described to you on initial meeting with Robyn and Veverly. If Robyn had described symptoms of left-sided hemiparesis at the meeting rather than both sides numbness in the extremities, would your diagnosis be the same? Mr. Jones: You are talking on the 1st? Mr. Mason, of migraines, on the 1st. A: Witness: It would have been --- it could have still been migraine but it would have changed the differential some. Q: The differential diagnosis? A: Yes. Q: Would it have moved Moyamoya higher up on the chain? A: No, but we would have done an MRI that day if she had weakness like that. (**My comment**: See his dictation of 10/05/2007.)

After reviewing all of these records, it appears that there is a discrepancy between what the family says and what the doctor's interpretation was. The family indicates that the patient never had headaches prior to October 4th, but only episodes of numbness, which are delineated in the deposition of the patient's mother. Dr. Garland's deposition is internally inconsistent with his dictation of October 5, 2007, in the hospital, indicating a headache associated with weakness on both sides of the body in the deposition, and a headache associated with left sided numbness and weakness in the dictation of October 5, 2007. In his deposition, he describes what a transient ischemic attack is and states that it is a subset of a stroke, and states that MRIs should be done in people who you think are having a stroke, and yet he contradicts himself in the deposition stating that her symptoms were not clinically an indication for a workup with an MRI. He makes a big distinction between symptoms occurring on both sides of the body verus only one side of the body, when in actuality transient ischemic attacks involving the basilar artery can produce symptoms on both sides of the body and are in effect a basilar arterial distribution transient ischemic attack and symptoms of numbness or tingling, or numbness, tingling and weakness on one side of the body can reflect hemiplegic migraine in a differential diagnosis versus a transient ischemic attack involving one side of the brain versus the other. Both of these scenarios, bilateral symptomatology and unilateral symptomatology, are still consistent with a transient ischemic attack and need to be worked up on an emergent basis.

Finally, after reviewing all of the medical records, it is still my opinion that the number one problem was that a 13-year-old female who presented to a neurologist with symptoms of transient neurologic dysfunction involving left face, arm and leg, of numbness and weakness, either associated with a headache according to Dr. Garland's October 5, 2007 dictation or not associated with a headache according to the family's deposition, or a headache associated with bilateral limb symptomatology in arms and legs, and prior to any workup being done, she was given oral triptan (Zomig). Oral triptan given in this scenario should not be used as it increases a risk of a stroke in patients with hemiplegic migraine or basilar migraine, even without an underlying vascular abnormality. Prescribing Zomig for Robyn Edwards was a breach of the

23

RE: EDWARDS, ROBYN
March 22, 2012
Page 8

standard of care and a substantial contributing factor to her stroke and its sequelae. This patient should have been admitted as soon as possible when the history was obtained on October 1, 2007, for workup to rule out a space occupying lesion or vascular abnormality, including an MRI of the brain and MRA of the brain (which does not require contrast) or other vascular workup such as an angiogram (which does require contrast), as well as other possible considerations such as sickle cell disease or other medical problems that could contribute to her vascular abnormality. If this had been done on October 1, 2007, it is within reasonable medical probability that her right middle cerebral artery stroke of October 4, 2007, may have been avoided. Given her history, by prescribing Zomig to Robyn Edwards after only one office visit without first performing a workup to determine an etiology was a gross deviation from the applicable standard of care. Because of this, the patient lost her best chance of having no neurologic deficit.

If I can be of any further assistance in this matter, please do not hesitate to contact me.

Date of this report is March 22, 2012.

Signed this 28 day of March 2012, in Orange County, California.

Sincerely,

David A. Lombardi, M.D.
Board Certified Neurologist
Qualified Medical Examiner

DAL:en

About The Author

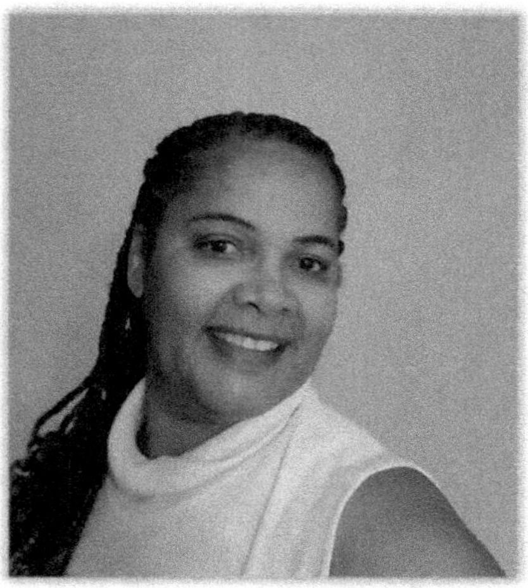

Veverly Myers-Edwards is a minister, educator, patient safety advocate, writer, and former consumer representative on the U.S. Food and Drug Administration's Neurological Devices Panel. She is the author of *God's Miracle Among Corruption in Idaho*, a documented record examining medical harm, legal failure, and the consequences when institutional oversight breakdown.

Her work focuses on medical accountability, civil rights, and the lived impact of systemic failure on Black families. She writes from direct experience, grounding advocacy in evidence, record-keeping, and public accountability.

www.ingramcontent.com/pod-product-compliance
Lightning Source LLC
LaVergne TN
LVHW052311200926
848481LV00002B/529
9798994775608